Quality Control Training Manual

Comprehensive Training Guide for API,
Finished Pharmaceutical
and Biotechnologies Laboratories

Quality Control Training Manual

Comprehensive Training Guide for API, Finished Pharmaceutical and Biotechnologies Laboratories

Syed Imtiaz Haider • Erfan Syed Asif

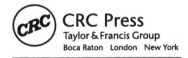

CRC Press
Taylor & Francis Group
Boca Raton   London   New York

CRC Press is an imprint of the
Taylor & Francis Group, an **Informa** business

CRC Press
Taylor & Francis Group
6000 Broken Sound Parkway NW, Suite 300
Boca Raton, FL 33487-2742

© 2011 by Taylor and Francis Group, LLC
CRC Press is an imprint of Taylor & Francis Group, an Informa business

No claim to original U.S. Government works

Printed in the United States of America on acid-free paper
10 9 8 7 6 5 4 3 2 1

International Standard Book Number: 978-1-4398-4994-1 (Hardback)

Visit the Taylor & Francis Web site at
http://www.taylorandfrancis.com

and the CRC Press Web site at
http://www.crcpress.com

To Mr. Saleem Riaz, the ex-Director of Quality Assurance, Abbott Laboratories, Pakistan, for his commitment to establish quality as an attitude in the pharmaceutical industry

Syed Imtiaz Haider
Erfan Syed Asif

Contents

Preface

Each year, graduates from community colleges to universities across the globe make excellent contributions to the pharmaceutical and biotechnology industries. Pharmaceutical science and biotechnology are now considered converging technologies that include nanotechnology, information sciences, and cognition, leading to massive changes in the nature of instrumentation, analysis, and manufacturing processes. Successful training solutions are needed to develop professionally qualified working environments in quality control laboratories in the industries in different parts of the world. It is estimated that nearly three out of four biotechnology/bioscience firms around the globe are growing at a moderate pace of 69%, including major expansions (9%), and holding steady around 27% in business activity levels.

Of the total business activity, 53% is attributed to those involved in clinical and technical work. A global review of the percentage of employees by job category indicates 30% work in production, 25% in quality assurance/quality control (QA/QC), 5% in analysis, and 3% in research and development (R&D). The average percentage rate of turnover by job function is 10% in QA/QC and 40% in production, which makes it most critical to fill the gap between experienced staff and recent graduates hired by providing in-house training before the latter can be considered qualified for daily routine operations.

General laboratory knowledge and entry-level skill techniques involve on-the-job training to accomplish routine operations in accordance with the good laboratory practice/good manufacturing practice (GLP/GMP), U.S. Food and Drug Administration (FDA), and International Organization for Standardization (ISO) requirements. However, the structured skills required for the entry-level technician in the therapeutic industry are verbal aptitude, recognition of symbols, pipetting, weighing, pH determination, aseptic techniques, clean room procedures, flow measurements, autoclaving, pressure measurements, molarity calculations, and the use of personal protective clothes, material safety data sheets (MSDS), columns, large-scale fermenters, spinner flasks, harvest equipment, and bioreactors.

The current work skills trend shows that 80% of the business industry believes that work quality can be improved 95% if industry-specific skills are provided in-house to entry-level staff, including appropriate evaluation and assessment.

A comprehensive quality control training manual guide for the pharmaceutical and biotechnology industry provides cost-effective training courses that involve the application of advances in the life sciences to produce commercially viable biotech products and services in terms of quality, safety and efficacy.

This book and its accompanying CD-ROM provide an administrative solution for management. The 17 training courses offered comprise detailed text, summaries, test papers and answers to test papers in both text and electronic forms.

The procedures can help companies to comply with GMP, GLP and validation requirements imposed by the FDA and regulatory bodies across Europe and around the world. The book also provides the FDA, Health Canada, WHO and EMEA guidelines directly applicable to pharmaceutical laboratory-related issues. The formats and styles provided are generic and can be further amended. The contents of the training courses are intended to build quality into the routine operations to comply with regulatory requirements. However, having a set of training courses does not preclude adverse inspection findings because the contents of the training needs that satisfy one inspector may not satisfy another.

We strongly believe that a facility's technical management and staff should avail themselves of these training procedures to ensure that particular needs are addressed with reference to the training needs of individual organizations and their regulatory requirements.

The ready-to-use training courses, in combination with the regulatory guidelines, provide a good source of training material for experienced and inexperienced practitioners in the biotechnology/biopharmaceutical industries.

The 17 training courses can be downloaded from the CD and adopted directly or after making minor changes. The ready-to-use test papers allow end users to record all raw data up to the issuance of the attached certificate.

The biotechnology/bioscience industries are regulated worldwide to be in compliance with current good manufacturing practice (cGMP) and GLP principles, with particular focus on safety issues. Each company is required to create a definite training matrix of its employees. The training procedures available in this book enable end users to understand the principles and elements of manufacturing techniques and provide documentation language ranging from the generic to the specific.

Compliance with FDA regulations is essential for companies intending to export their products to the United States. As a result, only a few companies are able to seek approval for export; one of the reasons behind this is the absence or inadequacy of the training. The training courses on the CD-ROM are valuable tools for biotechnology/biopharmaceutical industries that are in the process of developing training matrices to achieve FDA, Health Canada, EMEA, MHRA UK, WHO and GLP compliance. The training package is especially relevant to trainers, QA personnel, engineers, validation designers, internal and external auditors, technical training managers, and anyone interested in developing a qualification documentation matrix in the biotechnology/bioscience industry.

Acknowledgements

I am thankful to Dr. Ayman Sahli, the general manager of Gulf Pharmaceutical Industries, for always encouraging my professional achievements and continuously keeping me motivated.

I would also like to thank my colleagues and Taylor & Francis for their help in creating a professional environment. I am also indebted to my family for their patience while I compiled this book.

Syed Imtiaz Haider, PhD

It is a great experience to team up with Dr. Syed Imtiaz Haider and to create a new spectrum of pharmaceutical training manuals. My sincerest thanks to Dr. Haider for providing me his continued support and showing trust in me during another joint venture.

My special thanks to my wife, Dr. Beena Asif, for providing me the finest possible atmosphere for book writing, expressing deep interest in my work, and for her continuous encouragement in keeping me motivated. I would also like to thank my children, Rija Asif, Usman Syed Asif and Umer Syed Asif, for being around and still letting me do my work peacefully.

Not to forget that my mother, brother and sisters have always played a vital role in my successes by providing me moral support and making me feel their presence even from a farther distance. Their love remains deeply rooted in my heart.

Erfan Syed Asif, PhD

Authors

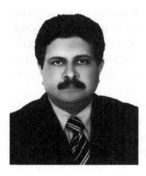

Syed Imtiaz Haider earned a PhD in chemistry and is a quality assurance and environmental specialist with over 20 years of experience in aseptic and nonaseptic pharmaceutical processes, equipment validation, and in-process control and auditing. Dr. Haider is currently involved in several major biotechnology-based tasks, including cell-line qualification, process validation, bioanalytics, method validation, biosimilar comparative studies, organizing preclinical studies, and preparation of the Central Technical Dossier (CTD) formatted for regulatory submission. Dr. Haider is the author and co-author of more than 20 research publications in international refereed journals dealing with products of pharmaceutical interest, their isolation, and structure development. A professional technical writer, Dr. Haider has authored more than 2000 standard operating procedures based on FDA regulations, ISO 9001:2000 and ISO 14001:2004 standards. He is a certified quality management system (QMS) auditor of the International Register of Certified Auditors (IRCA) and a registered associate environmental auditor for the Environment Association of Registered Auditors (EARA). He has written more than 10 quality system manuals for multidisciplinary industries and provided consultancy to the Drug Control Laboratory of the Ministry of Health in the United Arab Emirates in developing a QMS based on ISO 9003 and the later transition to ISO 9001:2000.

Dr. Haider works as a quality affairs director at Julphar, Gulf Pharmaceutical Industries and is involved in the preparation of several abbreviated new drug application (ANDA) files, which, after successful FDA, EU, and GMP inspections, will lead to the export of finished pharmaceutical products to the U.S. and European markets. He has also written *ISO 9001:2000: Document Development Compliance Manual: A Complete Guide and CD-ROM; Pharmaceutical Validation Master Plan: The Ultimate Guide to FDA, GMP, GLP Compliance; Validation Standard Operating Procedures;* and *Biotechnology: A Comprehensive Training Guide for the Biotechnology Industry.* Dr. Haider holds the intellectual copyright certificate of registration on an electronic documentation package on ISO 9000 and ISO 14001 from the Canadian Intellectual Property Office. He is also a contributing author of chapters on ISO 9001:2000 and ISO 14001 in international publications.

Dr. Haider has organized cGMP conferences in the region resourcing competitive speakers from Europe, Canada and the United States.

More recently, Dr. Haider has contributed to the Training Guide to Biotech & Pharmaceutical Industries and the *Cleaning Validation Manual: A Comprehensive Guide for the Pharmaceutical and Biotechnology Industries* with CD-ROM, published by Taylor & Francis Group/CRC Press.

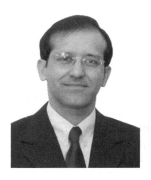 **Erfan Syed Asif** earned a PhD in organic chemistry and has expertise in various areas of quality operations with over 16 years of experience in pharmaceutical industries in Pakistan, the United States, Canada and UAE. He has worked in U.S. FDA– and Health Canada–approved facilities in different managerial positions. He has extensive experience in overseeing qualification projects for manufacturing equipment, utilities, systems, sterilization techniques, aseptic processes simulation, and sterile and nonsterile products manufacturing processes.

Dr. Asif currently holds the position of quality control manager in Gulf Pharmaceutical Industries, where his responsibilities include administrative routine in the quality control laboratory, investigating and responding to market complaints, advisory to production, introduction of new products, and conducting annual re-qualification of analytical instruments. Besides this, his role is to coordinate with QA managers to ensure GLP compliance in the laboratories as well as supporting QA in conducting external audits and inspections for the accomplishment of corrective actions. He is also responsible for overseeing the cleaning validation and vendor approval process and for conducting external audits of API manufacturers for Gulf Pharmaceutical Industries (Julphar).

As a validation consultant, he provided training and guidance on projects at Pharmacia & Upjohn, Michigan; Glaxo Smith Kline, Canada; and Air Liquide Canada (medical gas manufacturers) based on Health Canada and U.S. FDA regulations. He was also engaged in providing training on validation to various groups of validation consultants working on different projects in Canada and the United States.

Dr. Asif is the author of many research publications in internationally published chemistry journals and conference proceedings. He authored books with Syed Imtiaz Haider such as *Cleaning Validation Master Plan: A Comprehensive Guide for the Pharmaceutical and Biotechnology Industries* recently published by Taylor & Francis/CRC Press. He also participated as a contributing author having written three chapters in a book *Biotechnology: A Comprehensive Training Guide for the Biotechnology Industry* by Syed Imtiaz Haider and Anika Ashok, also published by Taylor & Francis/CRC Press.

He is also associated with the Director of Quality Affairs, Julphar in organizing cGMP conferences in the region and managing to gather competitive speakers from Europe, Canada and the United States.

Dr. Asif is a regular appointee of the Board of Advanced Research and Studies, Karachi University, Pakistan, as an external examiner for thesis evaluation and for conducting viva voce of MPhil and PhD degrees in pharmaceutical chemistry.

About the Book

This book and the accompanying CD-ROM take into account all the major international regulations, such as those of the Food and Drug Administration (FDA), the European Medicines Agency (EMEA), and the International Conference on Harmonisation (ICH) guidelines, as well as the industry standard ISO 9000, so as to be in compliance with training guidelines. No other book in print deals exclusively with training procedures for the biotechnology/biopharmaceutical industries or provides hands-on training aids that can be used directly or tailored to achieve training compliance in terms of good manufacturing practice (GMP).

This book is a good reference for entry-level technicians, managers, supervisors, and scientists in the pharmaceutical industry. The primary intent of this work is to guide manufacturing personnel and quality control professionals in the production of biotechnology-based active pharmaceutical ingredients.

This book provides exclusive training guidelines in a convenient electronic form on a CD-ROM to enable users to easily adopt them without losing time and achieve optimal resource utilization. The courses on the CD-ROM are valuable tools for biotechnology and biopharmaceutical companies that are in the process of developing a training matrix and organizing courses to achieve FDA, GMP, and good laboratory practice (GLP) compliance. The contents of each course are written in simple and precise language to meet FDA regulations and GMP and GLP requirements for training.

The book minimizes the number of documents that needs to be maintained for avoiding the nightmare of an FDA audit for the training manager. The procedures refer exclusively to the training skills required to achieve persistency in the quality control analysis.

The purpose of the book is to meet the need for a ready-to-use text on training in the biotechnology industry and to provide general information and guidelines. The concepts presented in this edition are not intended to serve as a final rule. Reciprocal training material for achieving this purpose exists and should also be reviewed and consulted, if applicable. The formats and style provided are generic and can be further amended. The contents of the training course are intended to build quality into the processes. Pharmaceutical, medical, and biotech industries are regulated worldwide to be in compliance with current good manufacturing practice (cGMP) and GLP principles. Each company is required to create a training matrix to qualify its personnel. The template training courses available here will enable end users to understand the principles and elements of specific skills. We strongly believe that the staff responsible for technical operations should attend these courses to ensure that particular needs are addressed with reference to operational control within the organization and individual country's regulatory requirements. The courses are guaranteed to provide management with a tool for developing a training matrix that can support a roadmap established for a successful and timely start-up in compliance with GMP requirements.

Compliance with FDA regulations by the health-care industry over the last decade has been a major goal, especially for those companies intending to export their products to the U.S. market. As a result, the FDA inspects several companies around the world every year for their GMP and GLP compliance. Only a few companies are able to seek approval for exportation; one of the reasons behind this is the absence or inadequacy of training programs in place. Key benefits of the book involve, but are not limited to

- Uninterrupted training
- Optimal training efforts
- Ready-to-use training text
- Ready-to-use test summary
- Ready-to-use test papers
- Ready-to-use test paper answers
- Ready-to-use certificate of attainment
- Training cost saving
- Marketing edge over competitors
- Improve company credibility
- Positive public opinion
- Improved training efficiency

We believe that by following the broadly based examples of the training topics, new as well as experienced companies can benefit by enhancing their current training approaches to meet FDA and other regulatory requirements. The book and CD-ROM are designed for individuals specifically involved in the writing and execution of training programs in the biotechnology industry. This book provides a complete, single-source reference detailing the basic training elements of the biotechnology/bioscience industry. The textbook on CD-ROM provides readers worldwide with resource data to train staff with varying degrees of experience at minimal expense without having to reinvent the wheel.

This quality control training manual has been organized as a database to instruct manpower involved in developing, manufacturing, auditing, and validating biopharmaceuticals on a pilot scale, leading to scaled-up production. Over the past few decades, there has been enormous progress in and substantial changes, additions, and enhancements of biotechnology in terms of the discovery of new biosimilars and their uses. Although different support documents, books, and research articles can be referred to for the principles of biotechnology and associated processing techniques, none of the books describe a single database with ready-to-use training tools that may require only minor modifications for customer convenience. The outlined training procedures have been derived from the basic principles of manufacturing biopharmaceuticals, from supported reference materials, and also from the personal experiences of the authors, who have been involved in the process of validation over the last 18 years in both pharmaceutical and biotechnology industries. Considerable care, thought, guides, and learning elements have been put together in this training guide.

We believe that this volume will serve as a valuable training reference guide that will be utilized again and again.

Disclaimer

Every effort has been made to ensure that the contents of this book are accurate and that recommendations are appropriate and made in good faith. The authors accept no responsibility for inaccuracies or actions taken by companies subsequent to these recommendations.

The similarity in the contents of the procedures, policies and guidelines—with a particular reference to the test functions, acceptance criteria and checks—may be incidental because of the similarity in principle.

QCT-01

Analytical Methods, Techniques and Quality Measures for General Pharmaceutical Products

QCT-01.1

Analytical Method Validation and Requirements

YOUR COMPANY NAME

Name: _____ ID No.: _____ Issued by: _____

Designation: _____ Department: _____ Date: _____

In pharmaceutical and biotech industries, method validation has received considerable attention from industrial committees and regulatory agencies and is applied to analytical procedures used for all dosage forms of products.

Analytical method validation can be defined as the gauges taken to prove that the analytical method employed for a specific test is suitable for its intended use, will consistently perform and produce results that consistently meet predetermined specifications. Quality control (QC) operations are by far the most important functions in pharmaceutical production and control. Therefore, a considerable portion of the cGMP regulations pertains to the QC laboratory and the testing of products.

As a matter of fact, the product's quality is very much based on the documentation, change control, validation and training of the analytical testing methods for evaluating products to and by laboratory personnel. Appropriate analytical procedures assure standards of identity, strength, quality and purity at the time of use by the public.

TEST METHODS AND STANDARDS

All the quality standards used by the laboratory should be complying with the United States Pharmacopeia (USP), British Pharmacopoeia (BP) or European Union (EU) monograph requirements.

If the in-house method is different from the pharmacopoeia, then the equivalency of the methods must be carried out and the availability of equivalency documents should be ensured.

TEST METHOD VALIDATION

1. A test method validation master plan must be in place supported by a general standard operating procedure (SOP) or method validation protocol for each product.

YOUR COMPANY NAME

Name: _____ ID No.: _____ Issued by: _____

Designation: _____ Department: _____ Date: _____

2. The method validation protocol must include, but should not be limited to, the following tests:
    i. Accuracy
    ii. Precision
    iii. Ruggedness (including site testing)
    iv. Linearity
    v. Limit of Detection
    vi. Limit of Quantitation
    vii. Range
    viii. Specificity
3. Each validation study must be in compliance with the product-specific protocol. If method is not a USP or another pharmacopoeial method, it must be verified to work in the lab.

TEST METHOD TRANSFER

1. The test method or technology transfer for new products from research and development (R&D) to the QC must be smooth and systematic and governed by the site policies and procedures. The method validation and method transfer reports should be available all time before preparation of standard test methods. Method transfer report includes
    i. Description of tests performed (or protocol)
    ii. Acceptance criteria (specifications)
    iii. Approval signatures by appropriate personnel

CHANGE CONTROL

1. All changes require formal approvals, including that of QA. A written procedure should be available, which prohibits making any changes except those authorized by QA.
2. Divisional and/or site policies and SOPs govern the control of any changes, which may affect product quality and/or regulatory commitments including changes in laboratory methods and/or controls. All such changes are governed by a system according to which the proposals, evaluation and implementation of changes in analytical methods could be controlled.
3. The change control system should be such that it provides a mechanism for determining whether the change will necessitate revalidation of the method.

YOUR COMPANY NAME

Name: _____ ID No.: _____ Issued by: _____

Designation: _____ Department: _____ Date: _____

For this purpose, the change control system must include a process of change evaluation by each concerned department including validation. In case revalidation has been deemed necessary, then protocol development and approval, evaluation and execution and scheduling and monitoring of the validation study should also be covered through a system and procedure.

4. The change control system should further require that a changed method be revalidated prior to the implementation of the change and release of product using the method.

QUALITY STANDARDS MANUAL

1. Each and every quality standard must be in the current revision status and must be in use. In order to maintain the document control, a list of approved current revisions must exist within the laboratory so that the analysts use the actual QSM while performing analyses.
2. The system to assure the current QSM revision must be in place, in the form of SOP. The same SOP may also be used to govern the official issuance of new revisions. The receipt and issuance of new revisions will then be logged in an appropriate logbook.
3. A periodic verification/reconciliation must be carried out to ensure the current status of all quality standards. To retrieve the old revisions of QSMs, a system should be in place.
4. The laboratory information management system (LIMS) must contain all tests listed in the quality standard including the proper revision of the QSM, and must be updated as per site procedure.

LABORATORY PROCEDURES

1. The laboratory must have an SOP for SOP. The SOP should also address numbering, issuance of binders and official copies.
2. The use of a new procedure must be prevented unless training on the procedure is accomplished and documented.
3. A system must also be in place to govern the current status of the SOPs as well as to ensure the regular review of all the SOPs in the lab. All such SOPs which are over three years old should be flagged. Historical copies of SOPs will also be maintained to track changes made over a period of time and, for the purpose of periodic maintenance.

YOUR COMPANY NAME

Name: _____ ID No.: _____ Issued by: _____

Designation: _____ Department: _____ Date: _____

TRAINING

1. Training should be effective. The measures for an effective training could be as follows:
   i. Assessment of outcome
   ii. Competency
   iii. Performance objectives
2. The effectiveness of training could be determined by assessing the proficiency of the trainee against a list of expected outcomes. The list of expected outcomes could be incorporated in the training module, designed for specific element of the laboratory. In case of failure of a trainee, a written action plan should be available to be followed.
3. A documented reinforcement training plan should include:
   i. Changes in cGMP regulatory requirements
   ii. New analytical methods or processes
   iii. New or revised departmental SOPs and/or Quality manuals
   iv. Atypical and out-of-specification (OOS) result investigations
4. In order to maintain the training record, documentation must be done that each analyst has received laboratory specific training, which includes training on specific methods and equipment. This may be maintained by assigning individual training file for each employee including managers, technicians, temporary employees, and so on.
5. Training files for each employee must contain the following information:
   i. SOP training documentation
   ii. Analytical methods/Quality manuals training
   iii. Analytical instrument training
   iv. All external training course materials
6. Mechanism must also be there to readily identify the analysts who are authorized to carry out each test method and operate each piece of equipment.
7. A documented formalized training program must be available to identify the specific type of trainings for the following type of laboratory employee:
   i. Managers
   ii. Supervisors
   iii. Analysts
   iv. Temporary employees
   v. Cleaners and clerks

YOUR COMPANY NAME

Name: _____ ID No.: _____ Issued by: _____

Designation: _____ Department: _____ Date: _____

8. The method of maintaining training information could be manual or electronic database. In case the training information is maintained in an electronic database, the system must be validated.

TESTING

1. All analytical testing must be conducted according to the written quality standards. This should also be reflected from the data recorded in the notebook that all requirements of the quality standards, for example, dilutions, equipment, columns and solvents, and step-by-step procedures are strictly followed.
2. In the process testing also the validated written procedures must be available, including established acceptance criteria/specifications.

RAW DATA

1. All raw data including calculations and test results will be recorded in bound and pre-numbered workbooks. The issuance and use of these notebooks will be controlled through a system and will be under the supervision of either lab supervisor or manager.
2. There must be an established system through which a thorough second check and review of all results and calculations will be performed on timely basis so as to assure the authenticity and accuracy of the data.
3. The raw data check system must include a careful examination of the following:
   i. Laboratory logs
   ii. Worksheets
   iii. Weighing
   iv. Dilutions
   v. Settings and conditions of instruments
   vi. Calculations
4. The laboratory data are to be stored under conditions that prevent damage from fire, water or other natural disaster. The raw data for all the tests should also be stored in such a way that they are readily available at the time of need. An SOP must be written and be adhered to in order to address the schedule for data retention.

YOUR COMPANY NAME

Name: _____ ID No.: _____ Issued by: _____

Designation: _____ Department: _____ Date: _____

CLEANING VALIDATION

1. Sampling and testing procedures must be validated before one starts using them for cleaning validation studies.
2. In order to support the cleaning validation analytical methods, recovery studies must be conducted to ensure proper sampling prior to implementation.
3. To ensure compliance in cleaning validation testing, training must be supported by the following measures:
   i. Attendance of the employee with number, title and department
   ii. Trainer's name and title
   iii. Date and venue of training
   iv. Duration of training (in hours or in days)
   v. Recording of results of training
4. All training records must be maintained at the allocated place according to the site's procedure and system (with QA or Human Resources). The procedure must also address the location's list if records are maintained at more than one place.
5. The review of training should be part of the internal audit.

RAW MATERIAL

1. There must be a system in place to assure that only approved vendors are used. In order to comply with this requirement, a procedure needs to be devised. The following are the measures to be taken:
   i. Established acceptance criteria
   ii. Certificate of analyses from vendors
   iii. Visual inspection
   iv. Analytical testing
2. Vendor's certificate of analyses must be kept in a file and should be accessible for review.
3. All raw materials including active pharmaceutical ingredients (APIs), excipients, and packaging components will be tested against established and validated test methods with pre-set acceptance criteria/limits prior to implementation.
4. In case QC lab has a reduced testing program in place then a procedure is required to describe as to when reduced testing can be instituted. According to the procedure, the reduced testing must meet all the criteria to support the use. In case one or more of the criteria are not met, the procedure must mention about the provision to revert to full testing.

QCT-01.2
Laboratory Equipment

YOUR COMPANY NAME

Name: _____ ID No.: _____ Issued by: _____

Designation: _____ Department: _____ Date: _____

Equipment is defined as an apparatus or piece of instrumentation in which testing or monitoring of laboratory samples (stability, finished goods, active ingredient and excipients, etc.) is performed. The precision and accuracy of these analytical instruments play a vital role in pharmaceutical industry to obtain valid data for research and development, manufacturing, and QC. As a matter of fact, developments in the automation, precision, and accuracy of these instruments parallel those of the industry itself. Regulatory agencies have certain requirements from pharmaceutical companies regarding the analytical instruments and their users.

Companies are required to establish procedures, assuring that the users of analytical instruments are trained to perform their assigned tasks and also to generate procedures, assuring that the instruments that generate data supporting regulated product testing are fit for use. The advent of qualification, calibration and preventive maintenance activities allows for laboratory equipment to continuously operate within operating parameters.

CALIBRATION AND MAINTENANCE

1. There must be divisional and site policies, guidelines and procedures available in the laboratory to address the calibration, maintenance, cleaning, change control and qualification of laboratory instruments, complying with cGMPs.
2. Care must be taken while establishing the policies and procedures for calibration and maintenance to handle both internal and external programmes. Mechanism for assigning tolerances and frequencies should also be a part of the SOP.
3. The SOP must also describe a control mechanism for changing tolerances and frequencies.
4. For contract calibration, the calibration and maintenance methods must be reviewed and approved by the company's quality system. The audit of

YOUR COMPANY NAME

Name: _____ ID No.: _____ Issued by: _____

Designation: _____ Department: _____ Date: _____

calibration and maintenance of contractors may also be conducted when needed. This must be outlined in the corresponding SOP.

5. Documentation must also show that the personnel performing the maintenance and calibration of equipment have been trained in the specific function they perform. For details in training, review Chapter QCT-01.1.

6. The QC laboratory or the maintenance department should have a master calibration list which includes all pieces of laboratory equipment that needed routine calibration. The master calibration programme may consist of automatic software that keeps all the necessary information about the equipment including the identity tag or asset number with the calibration frequency documentation.

7. Written procedures and methods for calibration and preventive maintenance for each piece of equipment should be available addressing the following:
    i. Schedule for calibration, maintenance and inspection
    ii. Responsible person/s for performing calibration and maintenance
    iii. Specific instructions for calibration and/or inspection
    iv. Responsible person/s for reviewing results and approval of calibration and maintenance of records
    v. Calibration tolerances and acceptance criteria
    vi. Requirements when a piece of equipment is moved

8. The records of calibration, preventive maintenance and inspection of laboratory equipment must be maintained appropriately in the laboratory and must be retrievable when needed.

9. The traceability of the calibration standards for each piece of equipment to a master standard must be presented in an appropriate document.

10. There is always a requirement from cGMP standpoint that all individual methods and procedures of calibration include a provision for remedial actions in the event—out-of-tolerance (OOT) situation is encountered. An evaluation of the impact on product is also required to be included.

DOCUMENTATION

1. Care must be taken in recording and documenting the usage, preventive maintenance and calibration of equipment. The laboratory logbooks may be used for this purpose.

2. Frequent checks of the logbooks must be performed to ensure that worksheets and electronic printouts generated from laboratory equipment

YOUR COMPANY NAME

Name: _____ ID No.: _____ Issued by: _____

Designation: _____ Department: _____ Date: _____

including qualification, maintenance and calibration are complete and accurate.

CLEANING

1. A written procedure must be available to provide instructions for laboratory equipment, glassware and utensils to be cleaned and/or sanitized at specified intervals. Such procedure should include the following as a minimum:
   i. Cleaning schedules and where appropriate, sanitizing schedules
   ii. Responsibility assignment for cleaning equipment and utensils
   iii. Procedure for dismantling and reassembling of equipment where necessary, to assure proper cleaning
   iv. Details of the methods, equipment and materials used in cleaning
   v. Proper inspection of equipment for cleanliness immediately before use

QUALIFICATION OF THE EQUIPMENT

1. The GMP requires the precision and accuracy of analytical instruments to obtain valid data for research, development, manufacturing and QC.
2. The regulations also require the companies to establish procedures, assuring that the instruments that generate data supporting regulated product testing are fit for use.
3. Ensure availability of a written procedure to address qualification of the analytical instruments. The SOP should outline the qualification status of each piece of equipment in the lab as well as identification criteria for qualification of each type of instrument.
4. None of the analytical instrument could be used without qualification. There must be a system in place, which may prevent the use of the non-qualified instrument.
5. Following the initial qualification, the annual re-qualification of the high-performance liquid chromatography (HPLC) units will be performed in house. All HPLC units will be re-qualified every year or as per the frequency established in the SOP.
6. The general SOP for installation qualification (IQ), operational qualification (OQ) and performance qualification (PQ) can be used to delineate directions for the qualifications of lab equipment as well. The procedure must also describe in detail the requirement of an approved protocol prior to commencing the qualification process.

YOUR COMPANY NAME

Name: _____ ID No.: _____ Issued by: _____

Designation: _____ Department: _____ Date: _____

7. The following tests must be carried out during the annual re-qualification of an HPLC unit as a minimum requirement:
   a. For auto samplers
      i. Linearity
      ii. Repeatability/precision
      iii. Carryover
   b. For pumps
      i. Flow accuracy test
      ii. Composition accuracy test
   c. For detectors
      i. Wavelength accuracy
8. The acceptance criteria for each qualification stage should be clearly outlined in the protocol. The execution qualification process must be according to the protocols. In case of a deviation from the protocol, a deviation report must be initiated with assessment of impact on qualification.
9. After the completion of a qualification, a report will be generated that must be in compliance to the protocol and approved by QA and other appropriate areas. All qualification reports should be maintained appropriately.

COLUMNS' RECORDS

1. A written procedure must be established to describe the steps and measures taken for maintaining HPLC and gas–liquid chromatography (GLC) columns' inventory.
2. A dedicated logbook should be available for inventory of the columns as per procedure.
3. GLC and HPLC columns need to be uniquely identified according to the book page number that contains a description of the column and notes its receipt.
4. Upon receipt of a new column with the test chromatogram, the chromatogram with the column number on it will be filed in the respective data binder.
5. The logbook must have the following information for each column:
   a. Manufacturer
   b. Model number
   c. Serial number
   d. Length

YOUR COMPANY NAME

Name: _____ ID No.: _____ Issued by: _____

Designation: _____ Department: _____ Date: _____

    e. Inner diameter
    f. Packing material type
    g. Particle size
    h. Pore size
    i. Date received
    j. Signature of receiver
    k. Any other comments—for example, description, and so on

COLUMNS' EVALUATION

1. Procedure must be in place, addressing the evaluation process of a new column of GLC or HPLC.
2. Evaluation of columns should be done in the following circumstances:
    a. When the column is being used for the first time in an analysis.
    b. If an equivalent column is used for analysis instead of the one mentioned in the standard test method.
    c. Every six months after the particular date, the column was used first.
    d. After any regeneration process of the column.
3. When the column is finally discarded, the reason behind this must be recorded in the logbook.

CHANGE CONTROL

1. All changes shall be governed by a change control procedure duly approved by QA. These changes may include but should not be limited to the following:
    i. Equipment or any piece of equipment: in order to assess if the change will impact the performance of the equipment and if a re-qualification of the system is required
    ii. Change to cleaning procedure of the equipment
    iii. Change to the maintenance and calibration procedures
    iv. Change to the calibration standards and frequencies

QCT-01.3

Reference Standards and Reagents

YOUR COMPANY NAME

Name: _____ ID No.: _____ Issued by: _____

Designation: _____ Department: _____ Date: _____

Reference standards and reagents are compounds, solutions and/or materials other than the samples themselves, which are used for comparative analysis of pharmaceutical products, or other samples (e.g., environmental samples, water samples).

The pharmacopoeia forums are routinely reviewed to assure that correct lot number of standards is in use. All USP or other compendial reference standards are ordered and received as per written procedure.

All reagents are labelled with the date of receipt, the date the bottle is opened and the initials of the person opening.

USP AND OTHER PHARMACOPOEIAL STANDARDS

1. A written procedure has to be established for ordering and receipt of USP or other compendial reference standards. The procedure should also describe the preparation (where appropriate) and control of primary standards.
2. Availability of correct lot of USP or any other pharmacopoeia standards can be ensured by routine review of the pharmacopoeia forum. A system should be in place for this process, which also provides instructions for ordering of these standards.
3. All the receipts for reference standards must be logged appropriately.
4. Only the current regulatory lot should be used. Upon receipt of a standard, the name, lot number and date received must be entered into the reference standard logbook.
5. Written procedure must also outline the need of periodical inventory check and documentation in a logbook to assure that only current lots are in use. Outdated lots must be destroyed.
6. The written procedures must also include provisions for prevention of contamination of primary standards.

YOUR COMPANY NAME

Name: _____ ID No.: _____ Issued by: _____

Designation: _____ Department: _____ Date: _____

7. The written procedures should specify all testing, including appropriate acceptance criteria, for all that must be performed on the standards.
8. The documentation for preparation and testing of all standards must be performed as per GMP guidelines.
9. In case an in-house transfer of standards is carried out between facilities, the procedure must be described appropriately in the SOP.
10. All primary reference standards must be stored under the recommended storage conditions mentioned either on the vial of the standard or in the safety data sheet supplied with standard.
11. The standard storage location should be secured, into which access is limited only to laboratory personnel having management authority.

REAGENTS, STANDARDIZED VOLUMETRIC SOLUTION AND BUFFERS

1. All the reagents must be labelled with the date of receipt, the date the bottle is opened and the initials of the person opening. The receipt and control of reagents should also be done according to a system described in the written procedure.
2. A mechanism needs to be established in the laboratory for ensuring that expired reagents are not used. According to this mechanism, the lab supervisor must keep strong vigilance to ensure that reagents are not used after expiry.
3. To keep a better control over the usage of reagents within valid dates, analysts must record the lot number and expiry date of the reagents while conducting a particular test.
4. There should be a system in place to assure reagent identification upon receipt and integrity throughout expiry and use. Tests for purity and potency, and so on could be used as for this purpose.

PROCEDURE FOR INTERNAL WORKING STANDARDS (SECONDARY REFERENCE STANDARDS) PREPARATION

SAMPLING

1. After the material has been identified as a potential internal working standard, sampling of incoming raw material should be performed for

YOUR COMPANY NAME

Name: _____ ID No.: _____ Issued by: _____

Designation: _____ Department: _____ Date: _____

characterization and certification testing. Sampling considerations should include, but are not limited to the following:

a. The material is fresh (not older than 6 months).
b. The intermediate container and packaging components are intact and are in good condition at the time of receipt.
c. No unfavourable, uncontrolled conditions occurred during transit, for example, exposure to excessive humidity or heat, and so on.
d. Appropriate documentation is included with the shipment, that is, dated purchase order and invoice, certificate of analyses including manufacturing date and data for all tests required as per pharmacopoeial specifications.
e. Samples are taken under laminar flow conditions into clean, dry, sterilized containers of adequate size and provided with hermetic seal. Samples are properly labelled and assigned an internal lot number.
f. The amount of sample is sufficient for all qualification tests and the quality of material is sufficient for one year's usage after such qualification.

TESTING

1. The samples of materials for qualification as internal working standards will be tested against current GMP standards.
2. The tests and specifications that are required to evaluate the suitability of the material, as an internal working standard must be defined.
3. As a minimum, the following tests will be performed:
   a. Description
   b. Identification (by more than one specific method)
   c. Moisture
   d. Purity or potency (any other applicable purity test impurities, degradation products)
   e. Any other applicable stability indication tests
4. The potency of each sample lot will be tested on an "as is basis" in triplicate, on three separate days, and preferably by the same analyst. This means that a total of nine tests per sample will be performed.
5. Evaluate statistically the results for potency/purity standard control procedures. If the individual results are valid, calculate the average value and assign the average potency/purity to the material.

YOUR COMPANY NAME

Name: _____ ID No.: _____ Issued by: _____

Designation: _____ Department: _____ Date: _____

STOCK SOLUTIONS, WORKING AND TEST SOLUTION

1. There must be a procedure in place for preparation and control of stock solutions. The procedure must also address how to assure stock solution's purity and potency.
2. The expiration dates set for stock solutions must be specified or the SOP should clearly state how many times as a maximum number the flask might be opened before the stock solution must be discarded.

EXPIRATION AND RETEST DATES FOR STANDARDS AND REAGENTS

1. A system should be in place and be described in a written procedure to ensure that replacement standards or reagents are ordered before their supply is exhausted.
2. A mechanism needs to be developed and adhered to which verifies that standards, reagents or solutions are in date prior to their use. This may be embedded in the same procedure described in point (1) above. The procedure must also address how the extending of the expiration date of standards, solutions and/or reagents will be carried out, in case the retest results are acceptable.
3. The traceability of the expiration date of standard, reagent or solution used for a particular test must also be ensured through a mechanism.
4. A procedure for safe disposal of expired materials must also be established and adhered to.

STORAGE

1. Storage of stock solution, reagents and standards is also critical. The storage should be done in a manner, which prevents contamination or degradation. This can be achieved by placing them in tightly closed containers in a cool, dry place. Protection from light or oxygen is also important where required.
2. All standards, reagents or solution must be stored under appropriate security, that is, in a locked cabinet or chamber. Storage conditions must also be strictly maintained as recommended for each type of standards, reagents or solutions.

YOUR COMPANY NAME

Name: _____ ID No.: _____ Issued by: _____

Designation: _____ Department: _____ Date: _____

LABELLING

1. All standards, reagents and solutions should have a standard label, attached to the respective container. The labels must include the following information as a minimum:
   a. Date of receipt
   b. Expiry date
   c. Date initially opened (for reagents)
   d. Identity
   e. Signature of person opening/preparing
   f. Purity (for standards)

QCT-01.4

Sample Management

YOUR COMPANY NAME

Name: _____ ID No.: _____ Issued by: _____

Designation: _____ Department: _____ Date: _____

Drug and finished pharmaceutical products sampling is a process used to check that a drug is safe and that it does not contain harmful contaminants, contains only permitted ingredients and additives at acceptable levels and that its label declarations are correct.

Because of the intentions to relate the results of analysis to the drug as a whole batch, it is crucially important that the sample is representative of that whole batch. The results of any analysis, therefore, can only be meaningful if the sampling is undertaken effectively.

Drug and finished pharmaceutical products manufacturers need to satisfy themselves that any sample taken for analysis is a true representative of the product for the analytical result to be meaningful. This is true whether the data are to be used as the basis of labelling declarations, assurance of compliance with legislative or other standards, monitoring of production as part of HACCP (Hazard Analysis and Critical Control Points), or for routine QC.

While inspections and investigations may precede sample collection, a sample must ultimately be obtained for a case to proceed, under the law. Proper sample collection and its identity, is the keystone of effective enforcement action.

Sample management represents the management of a process, as codified in various operating procedures, which concerns the sampling, identity, tracking, storage and retention of laboratory testing samples.

RAW MATERIALS, FINISHED PRODUCTS, IN-PROCESS, VALIDATION, SWAB, WATER, AIR, COMPLAINT

1. The sampling of raw and packaging materials and their retention has to be described in a written procedure.
2. A sampling plan must be established with scientific justification and statistical criteria such as confidence levels, component variability, degree of precision desired and the past history of supplier. These may be made part of another SOP.

YOUR COMPANY NAME

Name: _____ ID No.: _____ Issued by: _____

Designation: _____ Department: _____ Date: _____

3. The procedure must also address exact number of samples specified for various dosage forms, types of product and batch size, and so on.
4. Sampling plan should also include sample size and defined sample locations in case of powders, granules and liquids, that is, top, middle, bottom, and so on. These locations may be elaborated more if being carried out for validation.
5. The mount of samples taken must be sufficient for the quantity needed for analysis, retesting in case of OOS and retention as reference samples.
6. The sampling plans and changes, if occur, must be reviewed and approved by QA.
7. In order to facilitate tracking of samples, all activities related to sample flow should be performed as per approved procedure. These activities include sampling, sample login, storage, assignment to analyst, testing, documenting results, retention and finally destruction of samples. Samples have to be retained until documentation is complete.
8. Samples should always be done by specific and authorized personnel who are not only designated to pull samples but are also appropriately trained.
9. All sampling techniques for each specific product type must be addressed in written procedures. Sampling tools of different types must also be identified in the written procedure for samples for specific products and/or in-process bulk material. Sampling tools may be reusable, dedicated or disposable, however, should be clearly defined in the procedure.
10. Written procedures for cleaning of sampling tools should be validated and included in the cleaning validation master plan except for the ones which are dedicated or disposable.
11. Whenever necessary, sterile equipment and aseptic sampling techniques should be used for the sampling of raw materials or components.
12. While sampling care must be taken to avoid cross contamination of the materials. To avoid such incidents, containers should be immediately resealed after sampling. Materials, which are more susceptible to contamination, should be sampled in a controlled area.
13. Labelling must be done to all samples with the information as given below
    a. Name of material/component
    b. Lot/batch number
    c. Number of the container from which the sample was taken

YOUR COMPANY NAME

Name: _____ ID No.: _____ Issued by: _____

Designation: _____ Department: _____ Date: _____

    d. Name or signature of the person who took the sample

    e. Date of sampling

    f. Description of sample (e.g., blend, in-process, validation, cleaning validation, etc.)

14. The log book used in the lab for logging in samples must contain as a minimum the following information:

    a. Name of sample (sample description)

    b. Source of sample

    c. Date of sampling

    d. Quantity

    e. Analysis to be performed

    f. Date received in the lab

15. While sampling, all containers should be marked to indicate that samples have been taken from them.

16. All samples including the retention ones must be stored in containers meeting regulatory requirements and under specified storage conditions for temperature, humidity and light, and so on.

17. All samples for each lot of active ingredient must be stored within the specified time limits with controlled access to sample room.

18. The retention samples must be of at least twice the quantity necessary for all tests required to determine that the active ingredient meets its established specifications. All retention samples are to be retained for one year after expiry of the last lot of the product containing the material.

19. There must be a mechanism in place to assure accountability of retention samples.

20. In case the retention samples are opened and used to test for investigation or any other purpose, documentation must be done to indicate date/name of individual opening sample and reason for opening to keep the track of the usage of retention samples.

QCT-01.5

Stability Analytical Methods and Requirements

YOUR COMPANY NAME

Name: _____ ID No.: _____ Issued by: _____

Designation: _____ Department: _____ Date: _____

The main purpose of performing stability studies is to collect information regarding the impact that environmental factors such as temperature, light and humidity may have over the strength, purity, efficacy, quality and safety of drug substances and products. All regulatory agencies have emphasized on the significance of stability studies which makes it a critical component of GMP.

The following are the reasons based on which stability studies are considered important:

- Helps monitoring the product quality to ensure that drug products retain their full efficacy, quality, and safety up to the end of their expiration date
- Assures human health products meet appropriate standards at the time of use
- Supports post-approval changes
- Provides justification for recommended storage conditions, shelf life and stability testing frequency
- Helps to respond to customer complaints and possible recalls

WRITTEN PROCEDURES

1. An SOP must be available at the site to address the stability testing programme along with the presence of a stability protocol.
2. Once a stability profile is established additional lots of products are sampled following an approved stability protocol, monitored and compared to the profile on a continuous basis.
3. The stability protocol should address the testing schedule and plan in detail to comply with new drug application (NDA) commitments written for each product. Procedures must also define the sample size, test

YOUR COMPANY NAME

Name: _____ ID No.: _____ Issued by: _____

Designation: _____ Department: _____ Date: _____

> intervals and the number of lots to be tested based upon statistical criteria for each attribute to ensure valid estimates of stability.
> 4. The stability protocols will be pre-approved by QC, QA and product development departments. Any change in the approved protocol will require a further authorization by QA.
> 5. The termination of stability programme under any circumstances for any product also has to be included in the written procedure.
> 6. There must be a system through which the official SOPs related to stability studies are controlled in the laboratory. System should also discuss that the use of a new procedure be prevented if the documented training has not taken place. All the SOPs in the laboratory should be in the updated state and be reviewed on regular basis. Procedures over three years old can be flagged for easy identification and follow up.

ON SITE STARTS

> 1. In order to implement a successful stability programme, a procedure should be available to place at least one lot of each product/package on stability each year.
> 2. Furthermore, after each NDA or abbreviated new drug application (ANDA) approval, the first three lots, consequently the validation batches, must be placed on stability.
> 3. The changes in formulation, drug substance (supplier), raw material and container closure (sources), the manufacturing site or any type of reprocessing of material must be followed by the evaluation of stability data. The stability SOP should also have the evaluation process for the storage stability of bulk drug product.
> 4. The process change procedure may also include the time period as to when stability testing should be triggered.
> 5. In the solid dosage forms, the container sealant integrity is also challenged by stressing the adhesive properties. This is done by placing the samples on higher than 70% RH and 30°C.

TIME AND FREQUENCIES

> 1. All process change requests need a thorough review to ensure if the stability was conducted as indicated in change requests.

YOUR COMPANY NAME

Name: _____ ID No.: _____ Issued by: _____

Designation: _____ Department: _____ Date: _____

2. During the stability studies, the retrieval of samples should not be more than one week prior to the due date and tested not more than two weeks after the due date.
3. The stability protocol is required to clearly indicate that the testing is performed every three months over the first year, every six months over the second year, and annually thereafter.
4. If the accelerated study is performed as per protocol, testing has to be done on a monthly basis.
5. The time "zero" is defined as the first testing of the initial samples at the time of release. The initial samples are placed on stability afterwards and the time should not exceed 30 days after the zero time testing is completed. In case the 30 days exceeds, a provision to conduct another test should also be addressed in the procedure. The purpose of this second test is to equate this to time zero.

STATISTICAL CONSIDERATIONS

1. It is always a better idea to describe in the stability protocols what statistical methods will be used for analysing data.
2. Confidence levels should be calculated around the degradation curves, which should be based up on 95% of the label claim. The expiration data is usually based on the intersection of the degradation curve with the lower specification limit. However, if the product's stability increases with time the upper confidence levels must also be addressed.

EVALUATION OF STABILITY

The stability SOP in general contains the following considerations to evaluate the stability of a given product:

1. Provisions to ensure that current marketed containers/closures were used to pack the samples placed on stability.
2. Samples are derived from the lot so that they are true representatives of the lot/batch, which are selected without bias.
3. Samples for assay are taken from a new container each time, which means that the container was not opened previously. It is therefore suggested that a minimum of two containers should be taken for sampling.

YOUR COMPANY NAME

Name: _____ ID No.: _____ Issued by: _____

Designation: _____ Department: _____ Date: _____

4. For long-term testing, 25°C ± 2°C temperature is used to place the samples, with controlled humidity, which is generally 60% ± 5% RH. For accelerated testing, 40°C ± 2°C and 75% ± 5% RH is generally used.
5. The SOP should further address the requirement that in case a 5% potency loss or OOS condition occurs at 40°C, 75% RH, then a study at 30°C/60% RH must be initiated and continued for six months.
6. The SOP further includes the matrixing of the products based on sound statistical and scientific rationale.
7. In case extrapolation is used to assign expiration dates, a rationale needs to be required based on mechanism of degradation, goodness of fit of any mathematical model and batch size, and so on. All stability data must be evaluated on a timely basis including previous data points, as generated.

SPECIFICATIONS AND METHODS

1. The issuance and controlling of stability specifications should be under an approved system. Furthermore, the release and stability specifications must be considered together.
2. Testing requirements and standards: The testing requirements for various dosage forms and preparations as outlined in the procedure will be as follows:
   Tablet products: Tested for appearance, friability, hardness, colour, odour, moisture, strength and dissolution.
   Capsule products: The capsule will be evaluated for strength, moisture, colour appearance, shape, brittleness and dissolution.
   Solutions and suspensions: The testing parameters will be appearance, strength, pH, colour, odour, redispersibility, dissolution (suspensions) and clarity (solutions).
   For multiple-unit containers such as parenterals and aerosols: All sizes of each container/closure combinations should be placed on stability.
   Sterile products: Reasonable intervals must be outlined in the stability procedure for sampling and testing of small volume parenterals for strength, appearance, colour, particulate matter, pH, sterility and pyrogenicity. Injectables, which are intended for use as an additive to another drug product, will also be tested for the possibility of incompatibilities. In order to ensure container/closure integrity parenterals will be stored inverted or on their sides and then must be

YOUR COMPANY NAME

Name: _____ ID No.: _____ Issued by: _____

Designation: _____ Department: _____ Date: _____

tested for container/closure integrity at specific intervals throughout the stability study.

Topical preparations: All topical preparations will be tested for the presence of topical pathogens as part of the stability study. The ointments, pastes and creams in containers larger than 3.5 g will also be sampled and tested at the surface, middle and bottom of the container to ensure homogeneity throughout the shelf life.

Ophthalmic products: All ophthalmic preparations must be tested for appearance, clarity, colour, homogeneity, odour, pH, resuspendibility (for lotions), consistency, particle size distribution, strength and weight loss (plastic containers).

Metered-dose and respiratory inhalers: For metered-dose and respiratory inhalers, the specifications and testing requirements include delivered dose per actuation, number of doses, colour, clarity (solutions), particle size distribution (suspensions), loss of propellant, pressure, valve corrosion and spray pattern. The respiratory inhalants will further be tested for presence of *Staphylococcus aureus*, *Pseudomonas aeruginosa*, *Escherichia coli* and *Salmonella* species and total microbial count.

Suppositories: Suppositories need evaluation for strength, softening range, appearance and dissolution time at 37°C as per the stability procedure.

3. In case of drug products, both upper and lower limits of degradation products must be included. The major degradation products should be isolated, purified, quantified and identified under specific procedures.
4. In general, impurity profile is required to be generated, and if the impurities are at levels greater than 0.1% then they should also be identified. If for a drug with maximum daily dose of >2 g/day, impurities exceed 0.05%, then data must be acquired and evaluated to establish the biological safety of a particular impurity at the level specified.
5. The stability study protocol must address the requirement to ensure that preservative content of applicable drug products is monitored at least at the beginning and end of the stability study.
6. The stability system in place must further ensure that non-sterile products that do not contain preservatives are tested at specific intervals throughout the stability study.
7. There should be a provision in the site stability procedure to withdraw drug products, which do not meet stability specifications from the marketplace.

YOUR COMPANY NAME

Name: _____ ID No.: _____ Issued by: _____

Designation: _____ Department: _____ Date: _____

STABILITY METHODS

In order to ensure compliance with NDA commitments, stability methods must not be different from the documents submitted. In case the stability methods differ from USP, BP or any other pharmacopoeia, companies must perform the equivalency test and must maintain the documents to prove equivalency.

STABILITY METHODS VALIDATION PROGRAM

PRODUCT AND TEST-SPECIFIC PROTOCOL (V, D)

1. A general SOP or protocol for method validation has to be developed addressing the need of specific method validation protocols for each product.
2. The method validation protocol will include all of the elements of validation, which are as follows:
   Accuracy
   Precision
   Ruggedness (including site testing)
   Linearity
   Limit of Detection
   Limit of Quantitation
   Range
   Specificity
3. All validation studies must comply with the product-specific protocols. In case the method is not a USP method, verification must have to be performed in the lab before carrying out validation.
4. All methods have to be stability indicating.

TECHNOLOGY TRANSFER

1. The provision of site policies and procedures governing the transfer of methods is necessary. According to the procedure, the transfer of method for new products from R&D to the site should be smooth and systematic. The methods transfer documentation along with validation report must be present at the site for each quality standard method.
2. Generally, a method transfer documentation/report includes the following:
   i. A detailed description of the tests performed which could be either the specific test(s) or the formal approved protocol

YOUR COMPANY NAME

Name: _____ ID No.: _____ Issued by: _____

Designation: _____ Department: _____ Date: _____

    ii. Acceptance criteria
    iii. Approval by appropriate personnel including QA director

CHANGE CONTROL

1. For a change control in stability study, the same policy applies as for all other types of controlled documents that prohibit any change except those authorized by QA. The company's policy and procedure must govern the control of any change that may impact products quality or NDA commitments.
2. The proposal for a change in the quality standards, its evaluation and implementation should also be governed by a proper system at the site. This system will further evaluate if a revalidation of the method is deemed necessary after the change is implemented.
3. Once the revalidation has been deemed necessary, the system will require the generation of a revalidation protocol, execution and monitoring of validation study. The changed method will be implemented to release products only after successful completion of validation.

RAW DATA

1. As for routine testing, all raw data, calculations and test results for the stability testing are also recorded in either bound notebooks or pre-numbered work sheets. The control, issuance and use of such bound notebooks or pre-numbered work sheets should be done under appropriate system.
2. Comprehensive second checks/reviews of all results/calculations/raw data must be done on timely basis.
3. All laboratory data must be stored under conditions that prevent damage from water, fire, and so on.
4. The site procedure also governs the record retention schedule. This schedule must be in published form and be adhered to. Raw data for all tests conducted must be readily available.

TRAINING EFFECTIVENESS

1. The indicators such as competency, performance objectives and outcome assessment, and so on could measure training effectiveness for stability procedures.

YOUR COMPANY NAME

Name: _____ ID No.: _____ Issued by: _____

Designation: _____ Department: _____ Date: _____

2. Each training module should have a written list of expected outcomes that describes what the trainee is expected to learn or demonstrate knowledge of or proficiency upon completion of a training activity.
3. In case an analyst fails training, there should be a written action plan to follow.
4. There should be a documented reinforcement-training plan including new analytical methods, revisions in departmental procedures, utilization of new equipment and OOS investigations.

ANALYST-SPECIFIC TRAINING

1. It is necessary that all SOPs and laboratory-specific training received by each analyst is documented.
2. In case of critical analytical instruments, specific analysts may also be trained and be documented. In such cases, the documentation must also clearly mention that each specialized analyst has received specialized training. The procedure must also possess a mechanism to identify employees who are authorized to carry out each test method and operate each piece of equipment.

TRAINING DOCUMENTATION

1. Each type of laboratory employee must have a documented formalized training programme. The employees include managers, supervisors, analysts, temporary employees and support employees (glassware cleaners, etc.).
2. All the employees mentioned above must have a separate training file to log in the training results and other details. The file should contain as a minimum the following information:
    i.   Training on cGMP for new employee
    ii. Training on SOPs
    iii. Analytical methods training
    iv. Equipment training
3. The approved job requirements for each employee should also cross-reference with training requirements.
4. Training information may be maintained by electronic database or manual. However, in case of electronic database, system validation has to be ensured.

YOUR COMPANY NAME

Name: _____ ID No.: _____ Issued by: _____

Designation: _____ Department: _____ Date: _____

5. The following information will have to be presented in all training documentation:
    i.   Name, employee number, title and department of the trainee
    ii. Name and title of the person who conducted training session
    iii. Date, time, venue and duration of the training session
    iv. How training results were recorded
6. Records retention should be part of a written procedure. In general, it is human resource, which should be responsible for maintaining training records. A master listing of records location must exist if records are placed in more than one location.
7. The review of training records must be part of the internal audit program.

STABILITY CHAMBERS

1. The stability chambers are an integral part of the stability study. A procedure must be in place, which requires that stability chambers be qualified, routinely calibrated and monitored on a continuous or periodic basis.
2. In case stability chambers conditions exceeded for more than 24 hours the impact should be assessed and described in a written procedure including appropriate documentation of the event.

OUTSIDE LABORATORIES

1. Outside laboratory testing may be needed at times. A procedure should be in place where this need is addressed appropriately.
2. The procedure must clearly outline the circumstances when the need of testing outside laboratory is triggered along with the procedure to transfer the samples from stability storage area to the test laboratory.
3. There should be a mechanism to ensure that the outside laboratory tests the samples within the due time.
4. The procedure must also address if there is a special precaution required to protect the samples integrity, for example, prevention of product from freezing or avoiding temperature above 25°C, and so on.

QCT-01.6

Microbiological Methods and Analysis

YOUR COMPANY NAME

Name: _____ ID No.: _____ Issued by: _____

Designation: _____ Department: _____ Date: _____

MICROBIOLOGICAL METHODS AND TESTING

The microbiology department performs a wide variety of microbiological testing on active raw materials, finished products and packaging components. Besides this, the functions also include indirect activities such as the monitoring/testing of the environment, compressed gases, water and media control.

MICROBIOLOGICAL TESTING FOR NON-STERILE PRODUCTS

The non-sterile products discussed in this section are topical, inhalants, nasal solutions and raw materials.

1. All non-sterile products and raw materials of biological and botanical origin required to be tested for microbial limits. Microbiological laboratory must have a procedure to test the total number of microorganisms and to assess the absence of specific bacterial species.
2. There should be an SOP in place for validating the methods used. The validation document must be available when needed. The SOP for validation of microbiological test methods must also address the validation procedure of new products and new microbiological methods. The specifications for total count and specific bacterial species should also be outlined in the SOP.
3. There must be written procedures in place that outline the criteria necessary for rejection of batches of non-sterile product or raw materials based on micro testing results. Data will also be used for trending.
4. Companies must have positive and negative controls run with each test, where appropriate, microbiological testing methods must comply with NDA requirements.

YOUR COMPANY NAME

Name: _____ ID No.: _____ Issued by: _____

Designation: _____ Department: _____ Date: _____

GROWTH PROMOTION TESTING

1. The methods to be used for demonstrating the ability of culture media used in sterility testing and other microbiological procedures to support the growth of microorganisms are generally outlined in an SOP or standard test methods (STMs). The SOP must prevent the use of media before it has been approved.
2. It is also recommended to perform the growth promotion testing with organisms normally found in the environment of a specific site or a manufacturing location within a site.
3. The number of organisms used for inoculation of the sterility test media must be proper and documented.
4. All growth promotion tests must be recorded in separate logbook.
5. The media lot numbers must be referenced to the individual test results so as to keep the track of the media used in a particular test. A better idea is to keep a column of media lot number on each page of the pre-numbered logbooks for analysts.
6. The growth promotion procedure should also outline a system for the action to be taken if growth promotion test fails.
7. All the test organisms used for sterility test media must be checked for identity and purity.

MEDIA PREPARATION AND STERILIZATION

1. An SOP always governs media preparation and also provides instructions on how to sterilize media with a complete autoclave cycle definition.
2. Media should always be sterilized in qualified autoclaves. All autoclave runs must be recorded and charts are filled appropriately.
3. The autoclave qualification and cycle validation documents must be provided, when needed.
4. The following elements must be included in design qualification for autoclaves:
   i.   Exhaust system
   ii. No backflow
   iii. Appropriate air breaks
   iv. Steam supply
   v.   Pressure holds

YOUR COMPANY NAME

Name: _____ ID No.: _____ Issued by: _____

Designation: _____ Department: _____ Date: _____

    vi.   Initial jacket mapping study
   vii.   Routine cleaning of drains

5. All pressure and temperature gauges on autoclaves should be part of master calibration programme and be regularly calibrated. In case of a delayed calibration for more than a month than scheduled, impact testing would be carried out for the products released during that period and documented.
6. The approval, filling and change of temperature charts should be according to written procedure.
7. For the incubation purpose, the microwaves used in the laboratory should have adequate temperature and time control and must be regularly calibrated.
8. As for calibration, all thermometers and thermocouples used in the microbiology laboratory must be part of master calibration programme to be regularly calibrated.
9. Although biological indicators are used mainly for validation purpose, however, using them on routine basis is also highly recommended.

OUTSIDE VENDOR–SUPPLIED MEDIA

1. For media supplied by outside vendors, there must be a lot-numbering system in place.
2. All outside-vendor-supplied media should have expiration date on them and be subjected to growth promotion testing.

ASEPTIC TECHNIQUE TRAINING

1. The microbiology laboratory must have procedures describing the necessary aseptic techniques for microbiological and sterility testing. All new analysts should first get trained on basic aseptic techniques before performing testing.
2. Training must also be continued for experienced analysts on an ongoing basis.
3. A procedure should be established to evaluate the aseptic techniques of analysts similar to media fills on filling lines. This evaluation will become part of training documents. In case of failure in meeting the criteria, the analysts should be removed from the testing until they meet the criteria again.

YOUR COMPANY NAME

Name: _____ ID No.: _____ Issued by: _____

Designation: _____ Department: _____ Date: _____

GOWNING

1. The gowning facilities should demonstrate adequacy and must possess the following features:
   i.   Availability of step-over bench
   ii. Design of door handles for use without touching palms
   iii. Storage cabinets situated conveniently
   iv. The room air requirements as per FDA guidelines
   v.   Cleanable surface
2. There must be an SOP describing proper gowning procedures for sterility testing. All new analysts must be trained on this SOP.
3. The analyst's ability to properly gown should be evaluated by means of contact plate testing.
4. Analysts should not be allowed to perform sterility testing without successfully accomplishing the contact plate testing. The periodic evaluation then becomes a part of training. All test records related to analysts training must be documented.
5. The room cleaning should also be established in written procedures.
6. Persons responsible for cleaning must be trained adequately with the training documented.

STERILITY TESTING

1. Before performing a sterility test, ensure that
   i.   The testing environment and other controls are maintained consistently.
   ii. The method being used is consistent with commitments in the NDA.
   iii. The method has been validated to show that the product is not bacteriostatic or fungistatic as defined in the USP.
2. Manipulated negative controls should be used during each sterility test.
3. Care must be taken in samples incubation time, which should be for 14 days. Especially if the site's normal flora includes slow-growing organisms such as some type of yeasts and/or molds, appropriate amount of time must be used for incubation of samples.
4. Company must have a policy and procedure for investigating initial sterility positives for aseptically filled products.

YOUR COMPANY NAME

Name: _____ ID No.: _____ Issued by: _____

Designation: _____ Department: _____ Date: _____

AUTOMATED IDENTIFICATION SYSTEMS

1. Identification of automated systems in the microbiology laboratory is a significant part of laboratory processes. All the systems used should be validated as per a pre-approved SOP for validation of systems.
2. It is important that the validation be conducted with known laboratory contaminants. A protocol must be written and approved prior to validation with acceptance criteria outlined, for example, what organisms will be used and what acceptance criteria has the lab established for each identification. A control run must also be carried out with each identification load.

STERILITY TESTING FACILITIES

1. The facility and equipment used for sterility testing must comply with the commitments made in the NDA files.
2. The sterility test area must possess the following environmental parameters:
   i.   Test area has a class 100 environment.
   ii. The high-efficiency particulate air (HEPA) filters' integrity is tested on routine basis. The schedule must be available in an approved procedure.
   iii. Laminar air flow available.
   iv. Air velocity as per FDA guidelines 90ft/min +/– 20% at the work level. Positive pressure is maintained to adjacent, less clean area. Minimum number of air changes per hour must be documented if required.
3. Environmental monitoring program: There should be an established monitoring program for environmental parameters in the sterility test area, with specified alert and action levels. The alert and action levels specifications must be supported by rationale.
4. Cleaning and disinfection:
   i. All the cleaning and disinfection agents should be delineated in respective written procedure. The preparation for disinfection should also be part of the procedure.
   ii. The cleaning and disinfection procedures must be validated for their effectiveness on specific surfaces and on specific organisms as well as their recovery studies from surfaces. This could be incorporated with the cleaning validation programme of the company.

YOUR COMPANY NAME

Name: _____ ID No.: _____ Issued by: _____

Designation: _____ Department: _____ Date: _____

ENVIRONMENTAL MONITORING DURING STERILITY TESTING

1. Monitoring for viable airborne microbial particles must be performed continuously during sterility test. (Settling plates alone are not acceptable.)
2. To help establishing trend for viable airborne microbial particles, direct surface monitoring should be performed with replicate organism detection and counting (RODAC) impression plates and swabbing techniques before and after completion of aseptic manipulations. Same technique can be used for personnel monitoring before and after completion of each sterility test. The data tending in relation to products must be conducted on routine basis or as specified in the procedure.
3. A procedure must be established for review of number of false positives per employee or per product on routine basis. This would also set the alert and action limits and procedure to act upon appropriately.

WATER MONITORING DATA

1. Water is a significant raw material used in the pharmaceutical plant. Written procedures must be available to test each type of water used in the plant.
2. An SOP must be available to address the following requirements related to water testing.
   i. Current drawing of water system attached to the SOP
   ii. All sampling points identified and described as per drawing
   iii. Sampling techniques from each sample point addressed
   iv. Frequency of sampling and testing for each type of water
   v. Time requirements from sampling to laboratory for testing, if required
3. The current drawings of the water system must be kept updated as and when a change occurs.
4. There must be an SOP addressing the need to review and evaluate trend from the data. The SOP must further outline alert and action limits for each type of water samples and a system for follow up with corrective action.
5. An OOS investigation and corrective action SOP is an important part of quality systems. Procedure for handling OOS water-monitoring data may be integrated in the same SOP or a separate one could be initiated to handle the issues with water system.

YOUR COMPANY NAME

Name: _____ ID No.: _____ Issued by: _____

Designation: _____ Department: _____ Date: _____

6. The written procedure should also contain the following details:
    i. Established culture methods
    ii. Media used for culturing

COMPRESSED AIR FOR STERILE AREA

An SOP must be developed to describe the sampling and testing of compressed air used in the sterile area. The SOP should contain, as a minimum, the following details:

   i. Appropriate sampling techniques
   ii. Sampling points and frequency of testing
   iii. Training of personnel/s involved with sampling and testing
   iv. Schedule of testing and adherence to it
   v. Alert and action limits established
   vi. Mechanism for follow-up if limits exceeded
   vii. Trending of data and follow-up for any trends noted

NITROGEN TESTING FOR STERILE AREA

An SOP must be developed to describe the sampling and testing of nitrogen gas used in the sterile area. The SOP should contain, as a minimum, the following details:

   i. Appropriate sampling techniques
   ii. Sampling points and frequency of testing
   iii. Training of personnel/s involved with sampling and testing
   iv. Schedule of testing and adherence to it
   v. Alert and action limits established
   vi. Mechanism for follow-up if limits exceeded
   vii. Trending of data and follow-up for any trends noted

OXYGEN TESTING FOR STERILE AREA

An SOP must be developed to describe the sampling and testing of oxygen gas used in the sterile area. The SOP should contain, as a minimum, the following details:

   i. Appropriate sampling techniques
   ii. Sampling points and frequency of testing
   iii. Training of personnel/s involved with sampling and testing

YOUR COMPANY NAME

Name: _____ ID No.: _____ Issued by: _____

Designation: _____ Department: _____ Date: _____

   iv. Schedule of testing and adherence to it
    v. Alert and action limits established
   vi. Mechanism for follow-up if limits exceeded
  vii. Trending of data and follow-up for any trends noted

PRESERVATIVE EFFECTIVENESS TESTING

1. Test for preservative effectiveness should be performed through written procedure where the test methods are also described in detail. Care must be taken to ensure that the tests are performed as per compendial requirements whether USP, BP or EP.
2. Personnel performing above-mentioned tests must be appropriately trained.
3. The company OOS investigation SOP can be used to establish a mechanism to ensure compliance with compendial limits and to follow-up on any OOS results.

BACTERIAL ENDOTOXIN TESTING FOR STERILE PRODUCTS

1. Like all other tests mentioned in the lines above, a written procedure is also required to describe the test method used for bacterial endotoxin testing.
2. Personnel performing above-mentioned tests must be appropriately trained.
3. The company OOS investigation SOP can be used to establish a mechanism to ensure compliance with compendial limits and to follow-up on any OOS results.

QCT-01.7

Analytical Failure Investigations

YOUR COMPANY NAME

Name: _____ ID No.: _____ Issued by: _____

Designation: _____ Department: _____ Date: _____

LABORATORY INVESTIGATIONS

All results generated during analytical testing must be evaluated to determine if they comply with the standards given in a relevant specification or comply with defined acceptance criteria. If a result is obtained that is OOS or is considered atypical, a defined procedure must be followed to investigate the result and determine the course of action to be taken.

Laboratory investigations are documented assessments that are performed in the laboratory following an OOS or questionable result to determine if an assignable (laboratory-related) cause can be found.

The OOS results can arise from cause, which can be divided, into three categories.

1.1 Laboratory error
- Analyst
- Instrument failure
- Reagent problems
- Non-robust method

1.2 Non-process-related error
- Operator error
- Equipment failure
- Supplier error
- Sampling problem

1.3 Process related or manufacturing process error
- Non-robust process

YOUR COMPANY NAME

Name: ———————— ID No.: ———————— Issued by: —————

Designation: ————— Department: ————— Date: —————

OOS INVESTIGATIONS

1. The laboratory must have an SOP for evaluating OOS or questionable results.
2. The objective of the procedure should be to determine if the OOS result is valid, that is, the result is an accurate representation of the measured attribute of the sample taking into consideration, the precision of the analytical method and, if the result is valid, to determine the probable root cause of OOS result and its impact.
3. According to the procedure, upon finding an OOS result, the analyst must inform the immediate supervisor.
4. If the immediate supervisor is not available, SOP must clearly address what steps are to be taken in the interim period by the analyst.
5. It will be the responsibility of the immediate supervisor to assess the nature of problem and make a decision to inform the QC manager and production manager.
6. The analyst and lab supervisor are then required together to conduct a laboratory investigation according to established steps in the SOP.
7. When an OOS or questionable result occurs, there is a need to determine whether such a result is multiple (recurring) or isolated incident.
8. Laboratory investigation: The first stage of the procedure is laboratory investigation to determine if the OOS result is clearly assignable laboratory error. The recommended steps to conduct investigations include review of
   a. The testing procedure
   b. Raw data
   c. Calculations
   d. Preparation of standards and reagents
   e. Instruments calibration and maintenance records
9. Expanded investigation: If the OOS result is not clearly assignable to laboratory error, the next stage of the procedure is an expanded investigation, which includes provision for the involvement of groups outside the laboratory, retesting and, where justified, resampling.
10. The following points need to be considered during the laboratory investigations:
    a. Was the correct method used?
    b. Were there any deviations from the method?
    c. Were there any arithmetical errors in calculations?

YOUR COMPANY NAME

Name: _____ ID No.: _____ Issued by: _____

Designation: _____ Department: _____ Date: _____

    d. Was the equipment functioning correctly?

    e. Was the equipment calibrated?

    f. Were reagents, samples and standards prepared correctly?

    g. Should also consider non-assignable causes such as dilution errors and standard preparation error.

    h. Were the system suitability requirements defined in the method met?

    i. Were acceptance criteria defined in the method for precision of replication met?

    j. Was the analyst appropriately trained in the procedure? (Non-obvious assignable cause such as injection error)

    k. Were there any obvious physical problems with the laboratory sample?

    l. Were positive or negative controls satisfactory?

11. The SOP must also specify under what conditions re-tests should be conducted.

12. If the result of the initial laboratory investigation is inconclusive, a full-scale laboratory investigation is required. Tasks may include the following, if applicable:

    a. Re-analysis of the original solution (from the vial and/or original flask) to identify any equipment problems.

    b. Fresh dilutions from the original sample preparation or composite to identify dilution errors. At least two freshly prepared dilutions are required.

    c. New preparations of the sample to identify sample preparation errors. Three new sample preparations are required for each OOS result to demonstrate a root cause.

    d. Fresh dilution or preparation of the standard solution to confirm the standard response.

    e. Other defined tasks required to determine the root cause.

13. The initial retest must be performed by a second analyst three times using independently prepared solutions and a new instrument. A new composite sample should be prepared from the original laboratory sample.

14. Consideration must also be given for incorporation of the following aspects in designing the retesting procedure:

    a. A control sample is analysed as a part of the retesting procedure.

    b. The retesting procedure is conducted in two or more stages with a review after each stage (if the results obtained from the first stage

YOUR COMPANY NAME

Name: _____ ID No.: _____ Issued by: _____

Designation: _____ Department: _____ Date: _____

    confirm the original OOS results retesting can be terminated whereas if the results from the first stage are within specification or typical further retesting is conducted).

15. The procedure should also address the involvement of QA in the expanded investigation to determine the root cause for an OOS result.
16. The expanded investigation will include, but not limited to, the following activities:
    a. A review of the information available about the material under test
    b. History of the manufacture of the material under test
    c. Retesting where appropriate and justified
    d. Re-sampling where appropriate and justified
    e. Results of in-process testing
    f Results of other tests conducted on the material
    g. Review of training records of operators
    h. A list of other products and batches possibly affected
    i. The comments and signatures of all production and QC personnel who conducted approved any reprocessed material after additional testing
    j. The drawing of conclusions from the investigation, the assessment of their implications and the initiation of further actions as appropriate
17. At the end of expanded investigation all of the information that is available about the material under test (original results, retest results and data from the information review) should be taken into consideration in reaching decisions about the validity and significance of the original OOS results, the disposition of the material under test and the actions to be taken.
18. If the investigation has not identified the cause of the problem, investigations must continue as far as reasonably practical in an effort to determine the cause.
19. The SOP must also address rejection of batch and consideration to the following:
    a. Corrective action to prevent recurrence
    b. Implications for other batches of the same material and batches of other materials
20. In case the batch proves to be compliant as a result of retesting, specific directives must be present for disposition of batch.
21. As per the procedure, all the samples and reagents will be retained until the investigation has been completed.

YOUR COMPANY NAME

Name: _____ ID No.: _____ Issued by: _____

Designation: _____ Department: _____ Date: _____

22. The SOP should also define a system to inform upper management when OOS or questionable result investigations are being conducted and to make them aware of the conclusions.
23. The conclusions reached and actions taken must be documented in a final report and approved by QC, production (if failure is related to manufacturing process) and QA as a final approval authority.
24. The raw data and the results of all analytical testing and retesting performed on a sample must be retained in the laboratory records. This includes the data for the initial test in stations where laboratory error is proven.

TRAINING ON OOS PROCEDURE

1. The effectiveness of training on OOS investigations procedure must be measured by competency and performance objectives of the individuals.
2. Each analyst must go through the training on OOS SOP.
3. The SOP writers must also be trained with training documented.
4. There must be a written list of expected results for each training module that describes what the analyst is expected to learn upon completion of a training activity.
5. In case of a failure in training, a written action plan must be available to be followed.
6. There must be a mechanism to identify employees who are authorized to carry out OOS investigations. Preferably an authorized analyst should be used to conduct OOS investigations.

TRAINING DOCUMENTATION

1. For each type of laboratory employee a documented formalized training programme must be available. The SOP training documentation must also be available in the employees training file.
2. Type of employees is as follows:
   a. Managers
   b. Supervisors
   c. Analysts (temporary and permanent)
3. All the training information must be maintained appropriately. A validated electronic database is preferable, though.

YOUR COMPANY NAME

Name: _____ ID No.: _____ Issued by: _____

Designation: _____ Department: _____ Date: _____

4. The training documentation must contain the following as a minimum:
   a. Name of attendee
   b. Employee or ID number
   c. Title of attendee
   d. Department
   e. Name of the instructor
   f. Date and time of training
   g. Duration of training session (hours and days)
   h. Training records
5. The HR or QA department should be responsible for maintaining the training records. The retention of records must be a part of written procedure with clear indication of the location of records. In case of more than one location, there should be a master list of all locations attached with the written procedure.

QCT-01.8

Calibration Program

YOUR COMPANY NAME

Name: _____ ID No.: _____ Issued by: _____

Designation: _____ Department: _____ Date: _____

At the simplest level, calibration is a comparison between measurements—one of known magnitude or correctness made or set with one device and another measurement made in as similar a way as possible with a second device. The calibration process begins with the design of the measuring instrument that needs to be calibrated. The design must be able to "hold a calibration" through its calibration interval. In other words, the design has to be capable of measurements that are "within engineering tolerance" when used within the stated environmental conditions over some reasonable period of time.

In pharmaceutical QC laboratories, an instrument is considered to be properly calibrated as long as it returns values that are within predetermined specifications when compared against known quantities.

QC laboratories should ensure that analytical instrument, including mechanical, electronic, automated, chemical or other equipment, are

- Suitable for the intended use in the design, manufacture and testing of components
- Capable of producing valid and reproducible results
- Operated by trained and experienced analysts
- Properly calibrated versus a suitable standard

To succeed, the quality system shall include a calibration program that is at least as stringent as that required by the QS regulation (820.72). The intent of the GMP calibration requirements is to assure adequate and continuous performance of measurement equipment with respect to accuracy and precision, and so on.

QC INSTRUMENTS CALIBRATION

1. Written procedures must be established to conduct calibration of all critical instruments/systems associated with equipment in QC and

YOUR COMPANY NAME

Name: _____ ID No.: _____ Issued by: _____

Designation: _____ Department: _____ Date: _____

microbiology laboratories that is GMP related and used in control for the testing of drug products.

2. All these instruments/equipment must be calibrated and re-qualified at predetermined intervals by appropriate methods to ensure that they are capable of fulfilling their intended use. The intervals of testing are to be defined in the calibration plan.

3. A master calibration plan must be initiated by the plant's maintenance department, which should also include all instruments used in the QC laboratory.

4. When a new instrument is included in QC lab, a request should be initiated by the laboratory manager or supervisor for maintenance department to log in the new system/instrument in the calibration master plan to ensure regular monitoring of calibration.

5. The procedure must also address that QC department will be responsible for ensuring the availability of the instrument for calibration according to the schedule.

6. The master schedule should contain the following information of the system as a minimum:
   a. **System ID**—describes the ID number of the system/equipment
   b. **Description**—name of the system
   c. **Equipment type/status**—for example, HPLC
   d. **Location**—in which lab the system is located; for example, instrument room, chemical lab, and so on
   e. **Serial number**—serial number of the system
   f. **Frequency**—the frequency with which the system is required to be re-qualified or calibrated, whichever applicable
   g. **Procedure**—requirement for the system; for example, re-qualification or calibration
   h. **Book no.**—the number of file, which contains the calibration reports of the corresponding system
   i. **Due date**—the next due date for calibration, which is calculated automatically by the software

CALIBRATION PROCEDURE

1. Each calibration procedure must be described in detail in separate SOP, specifically written for a particular instrument/system of the laboratory.

YOUR COMPANY NAME

Name: _____ ID No.: _____ Issued by: _____

Designation: _____ Department: _____ Date: _____

2. A typical equipment calibration procedure must include at least the following:
   a. Purpose and scope
   b. Frequency
   c. Equipment and standards required
   d. Limits for accuracy and precision
   e. Preliminary examinations and operations
   f. Calibration process description
   g. Remedial action for product
   h. Documentation requirements

CALIBRATION FREQUENCY

1. The SOP must also address that the calibration frequency for each instrument, provided by the manufacturer, should be included in the calibration procedure of the particular instrument.
2. This frequency is then added to the master calibration program, which must be adhered to unless a change is deemed necessary. However, if any change in an equipment takes place, all the instruments associated with it will be calibrated before reusing the system regardless of the next calibration due date of the respective instrument.
3. Any instrument, that is removable for calibration will be removed by the QC department's personnel and handed over to maintenance department after official notification by QC. After completion of calibration the equipment shall be returned to the laboratory.
4. At the due date, it is required according to the procedure that the QC laboratory co-coordinator or manager follow up and make sure that the calibration is performed on time and accurately. They also will ensure that the calibration report is completed properly. The QC department will keep the calibration record in the corresponding binder, marked for the specific piece of equipment/instrument.
5. In case an equipment/system has passed due date for calibration, a "Do not use/Out of calibration" sticker must be immediately placed on it by the laboratory supervisor or manager. The equipment/system must not be used unless re-qualified/calibrated.
6. Clear instructions must be added to the procedure as to how QA will assess the impact on products quality if an out-of-calibration instrument is accidently used in the analysis and will document it.

YOUR COMPANY NAME

Name: _____ ID No.: _____ Issued by: _____

Designation: _____ Department: _____ Date: _____

7. The calibration SOP must also define the necessary actions to be taken
   in case a non-scheduled calibration comes up. Under such circumstances
   the equipment/system owner must inform the maintenance department
   or the calibration coordinator, in written, about the requirement and
   request to perform calibration.
8. The calibration coordinator will follow up and make sure that the calibration is performed accurately. Proper completion of calibration record
   will also be ensured. Calibration master plan will then be updated
   accordingly.

DOCUMENTATION

The calibration report signed off by QC and maintenance managers will be kept
as record in the calibration document room and will be maintained by the maintenance department. A copy of the same may also be kept in the QC documents
archive room for reference.

QCT-01.9

Laboratory Facility

YOUR COMPANY NAME

Name: _____ ID No.: _____ Issued by: _____

Designation: _____ Department: _____ Date: _____

The area used for analysing, holding and retention of raw/packaging material, bulk/in-process, finished products and stability samples should be of suitable design, size, construction and location, environmental conditions, housekeeping and personnel practices to facilitate cleaning, maintenance and proper operations, which are necessary for conducting the required laboratory testing or that may affect the conduct of such testing or may put the quality of samples under jeopardy.

GENERAL REQUIREMENTS

1. Adequate space should be available for the orderly placement of analytical instrument to avoid congestion and mix-up of test samples of different materials and products.
2. There should be defined area for each analyst according to the nature of his/her work. The design of the test facility must provide an adequate degree of separation of the different activities to assure the proper conduct of testing.
3. The laboratory must have a separate area for storage of samples, which are to be tested, or are under testing. Care must be taken in keeping the samples segregated to avoid unnecessary repetition of work. The storage areas must be adequately protected against infestation and contamination. In general, the following areas or controls should be defined in the laboratory as per the following activities:
   a. Room for receiving and storage of samples before testing; this includes allocated areas for raw, packaging materials, sterile, non-sterile, in-process, finished, retention file samples, and so on.
   b. Instrument room where all HPLC and gas chromatography (GC) instrument may be located.
   c. Chemical room to conduct conventional testing as well as dissolution, disintegration and other photospectrometric analyses.

YOUR COMPANY NAME

Name: _____ ID No.: _____ Issued by: _____

Designation: _____ Department: _____ Date: _____

    d. Physical test room.
    e. Microbiology laboratory to conduct microbiological analyses.
    f. Sterility room specifically designed to conduct sterility assurance test.
    g. Sufficient space in the microbiology laboratory to install adequate number of laminar flow hoods.
    h. Area for keeping autoclaves, incubator and ovens for microbiology purpose.
    i. Refrigeration provided for perishable samples or selected test systems.
4. Adequate lighting should be provided in all areas of laboratory to facilitate proper functioning.
5. Ventilation in the laboratory must be adequate to provide appropriate working atmosphere for the analysts.
6. Equipment for the control and monitoring of air pressure, microorganisms, dust, humidity and temperature should also be provided especially for the microbiological laboratory.
7. Potable water should be supplied under continuous positive pressure in a plumbing system free from defects. Potable water should meet the standards prescribed in the Environmental Protection Agency's Primary Drinking Water.

AREA FOR HANDLING TEST AND REFERENCE SUBSTANCES

1. To prevent contamination or mix-ups, separate areas for the receipt and storage of the reference and test substances must be allocated.
2. The storage areas should be adequate to maintain the identity, concentration, purity and stability of the test substances.
3. Area to provide safe storage for hazardous materials must also be provided.

AREAS FOR ROUTINE SAMPLES AFTER COMPLETE TESTING

1. A written procedure must be established to address handling of remaining samples after testing. As per the procedure, all remaining samples after complete analyses will be treated as "pharmaceutical waste."
2. A separate room or area must be allocated for remaining samples of all dosage forms. Liquid products will be discarded in drainage system,

YOUR COMPANY NAME

Name: _____ ID No.: _____ Issued by: _____

Designation: _____ Department: _____ Date: _____

while empty label bottles will also be treated as "pharmaceutical waste."

3. Dry products and remaining packaging material will be put in plastic trash bags or carton boxes labelled clearly, "pharmaceutical waste," transferred to the pharmaceutical waste area from where it will be transferred to the municipality people to pick up and dump.

REFERENCE SAMPLES AFTER EXPIRY

1. There must be a procedure in the laboratory, which describes the procedure of discarding the reference samples after expiry.
2. Separate area must be specified for this purpose with a computer and access to database to show the expiry of batches from the reference samples. The details of expired reference sample should be entered to a designated logbook.
3. All samples will then be treated as pharmaceutical waste as mentioned in the lines above.

ARCHIVE ROOM

1. An archive room for the storage and retrieval of raw data, reports and samples should be available either in the same laboratory or in a satellite facility. Adequate space must be provided for the archive room.
2. Samples of raw and packaging materials and finished products should be arranged in serial numbers according to the batch number for easy tracking. All commodities will be kept separately though.
3. Ensure availability of temperature and humidity recorder in the room, with strict adherence to the calibration program for the recorder. The temperature and humidity readings must be monitored on daily basis and recorded in a logbook.
4. The archive room's space must be adequate to accommodate samples to be retained one year after the expiry date for finished products and 3 years for the raw materials.
5. Adequate monitoring must be performed for the premises where retention and stability samples are housed. There must be controlled access to these areas. Ideally, a logbook should be maintained to check and control the entry of personnel in these areas.

YOUR COMPANY NAME

Name: ——————————— ID No.: ——————————— Issued by: —————————

Designation: ——————————— Department: ——————————— Date: ———————————

STORAGE OF BACTERIAL STRAINS

1. The written procedure must be established for the proper storage of bacterial strains so as to minimize loss of viability.
2. To reduce change in culture, a seed stock should be established from the early passage cells.
3. This may be accomplished by propagating the strain under ideal conditions, by using the recommended medium, atmosphere and temperature.

CLEANING, DISINFECTING AND WASHING GLASS APPARATUS

1. Procedures must be available for routine cleaning of laboratories, washing of laboratory apparatus and disposal of broken glassware.
2. The cleaning procedures should clearly detail the differences between housekeeping and laboratory analysts' responsibilities. The housekeeping personnel should not be touching samples or any items on lab benches.
3. Cleaning personnel conducting cleaning should be trained in appropriate procedures.
4. The laboratory should be cleaned at least once a week and the floors should be swept at least twice a week.
5. Microbiological area:
   a. The microbiological areas must be cleaned with 5% sodium hypochlorite (1:8 dilution) before and after finishing each shift in the lab.
   b. Solution of 3% H_2O_2 should also be used to disinfect the working surfaces at least once a week.
   c. Dedusting must also be done in microbiology lab for windows, tables, chairs, walls, doors, roof and false ceiling, AC exhaust and cabinets, and so on.
   d. For cleaning sterility testing room, only freshly prepared solutions and disinfectants should be used.
   e. Disinfect the prepared media before passing them in the clean rooms using approved sanitizer.
   f. Care must be taken not to damage HEPA filters by direct spray of sanitizer.
6. Incubators and refrigerators: Incubators and refrigerators in the microbiology lab must be cleaned as per the procedure once a month, whereas in the chemical lab, cleaning of these equipments should be done once in

YOUR COMPANY NAME

Name: _____ ID No.: _____ Issued by: _____

Designation: _____ Department: _____ Date: _____

3 months. Disinfection of incubators and refrigerators should be done by using 70% ethyl alcohol or 3% H_2O_2.

7. Laboratory glassware should be washed by hands. Glassware are first rinsed with sanitary water, and then washed with liquid soap by means of a sponge or special brush as per the shape of the glassware. When required, chromic acid cleansing mixture (Ref. USP 30) should be used, and should then be rinsed thoroughly. Finally, rinsing should be done with deionized water.

UTILITIES

1. The type of water required in the laboratory must be clearly defined. The site's water monitoring program should also include points related to use of water in the laboratory.
2. The written procedure must also contain the action plan in case an OOS water result is obtained for a laboratory sampling point.
3. An action plan must also be outlined for electricity failure in emergencies.
4. Handling procedure should detail the action/s taken for the tests, which were in progress subsequent to emergencies.

SAFETY SHOWER

1. The labs must be equipped with a safety shower installed near the door.
2. To ensure proper functioning, the shower must be checked periodically, preferably every week.
3. Checking of the safety shower must be entered into a logbook with date and signature of the person responsible for checking the performance.
4. The outlet of the safety shower should also be cleaned frequently to ensure that there is no blockage in the outlet.

QCT-01.10

Products Annual Reviews

YOUR COMPANY NAME

Name: _____ ID No.: _____ Issued by: _____

Designation: _____ Department: _____ Date: _____

ANNUAL REVIEWS

Annual product reviews process is established to determine the need for changes in drug products specifications, manufacturing procedures of collecting and reviewing critical types of information, such as, product potency, complaints, stability data and deviations, to show trends and to discover any unusual or unexpected events, in order to determine the need for changes in drug product specifications or manufacturing or control procedures.

WRITTEN PROCEDURES

1. The site must develop and adhere to the SOP for annual product reviews detailing all required information and evaluation elements. The procedure should comply with 21 Code of Federal Regulations (CFR), part 211.180, as well as EU GMP guidelines.
2. As per the SOP, the following areas should be included in the annual review:
   a. Complaints (marketing and QC)
   b. Stability test results (QC)
   c. Recalls and rejections (QA)
   d. OOS and investigations (QC, QA and production)
   e. Finished product test results (QC)
   f. Manufacturing process description
   g. Process capability review (QA)
   h. In-process test results (QA/QC)
   i. Laboratory test results (QC)
   j. Process change requests (production, product development and QA)
   k. Analytical methods and quality standards change requests (QC and product development)
   l. Equipment/systems/facilities change requests (maintenance)
   m. Conditional releases (QC and QA)

YOUR COMPANY NAME

Name: _____ ID No.: _____ Issued by: _____

Designation: _____ Department: _____ Date: _____

    n. Atypical and abnormality reports
    o. Qualification/validation studies (validation, maintenance and QA)
    p. Quarantines (stores)
    q. Returned goods (stores)
    r. Salvaged products
    s. Component quality
    t. Annual examination of retention samples

3. The SOP must also describe the responsibilities for conducting the review. For example, QA, QC, product development and computer departments are usually involved in the provision and compilation of data.

4. A timeline needs to be established for the completion of annual reviews. Generally, the reviews will have to be completed within 60 days of the anniversary of its NDA/ANDA submission or campaign completion date.

5. SOP must clearly outline as to how the review will be conducted; whether it requires the review of data from a representative number of lots manufactured during the review period or each and every lot manufactured and released during the period, needs to be addressed.

6. Critical data for both manufacturing intermediates and finished product should be collected, accurately transcribed, analysed and compared to the corresponding specifications.

MANAGEMENT REVIEW

7. Annual reviews should include an executive summary of the product manufacturing experience during the review period. Each subsequent year a collective report based on quantitative and qualitative results of all test—physical, chemical, microbiological—will be printed for each product.

8. The appropriate management from manufacturing, technical services/operations, QC, and validation departments must review these annual reviews. Tools to detect trending will also be employed including use of graphical representation of test results and specification limits.

9. All these review inputs and comments along with any corrective action should be included in the form and attached with the finished product reports. The review conclusion must not be delayed more than the first quarter of the next year.

YOUR COMPANY NAME

Name: _____ ID No.: _____ Issued by: _____

Designation: _____ Department: _____ Date: _____

10. QA manager will forward final reports requiring corrective actions to the respective departments for implementing the changes.
11. Quality affair's director will finally approve all the reports. QA will retain all records related to annual product review.

DATA RELIABILITY

1. A second check should always be performed on data transcribed as part of annual review data gathering.

USE OF ONGOING STATISTICS

1. Ongoing data capture, trending and statistical analysis must be carried out on an ongoing basis.
2. Procedure must emphasize on establishing upper and lower control limits.
3. Statistical evaluation of the data must be performed in each annual review. The conclusions are drawn by the appropriate level of personnel and then documented.

FOLLOW-UP

1. There must be clear guidelines in the written procedure for further investigations if anomalies are found in any of the data reviewed or in the resulting analysis.
2. Procedure should also be established for assuring that recommendations made in annual reviews are acted upon.
3. Follow-up should also be documented for the annual review recommendations.

QCT-01.11

Third-Party Testing

YOUR COMPANY NAME

Name: _____ ID No.: _____ Issued by: _____

Designation: _____ Department: _____ Date: _____

Health regulatory agencies in the United States recall hundreds of products each year to prevent injury to customers. Product failures may occur as a result of flaws in drug designing, defects in manufacturing processes, tampering, or failure to meet safety standards.

Companies involved in a product recall have to face a series of impacts and need to take a number of corrective actions, which may include changing product design and packaging, withdrawing products from the distribution channels, announcing the product hazards to the public, as well as offering replacements to the affected.

Product recalls can often be prevented through third-party product testing. Third-party testing normally occurs before any significant manufacturing has taken place. The most preferable time is while a product is in the design stage. The potential problem areas can be detected prior to the production process and before the product is available for commercial use.

Third-party testing is critical to the detection and elimination of defects, before users ever experience them. The third-party testing provides an independent check and balance to ensure that the QC laboratory or outsourcer is delivering a product that will not surprise and frustrate its users at a later time. However, this may not be the only reason for a laboratory to outsource its activities. Many laboratories often do not have the resources or expertise required to conduct a certain type of analysis. Under such circumstances, an alternate site or an external contractor-performing laboratory testing (physical measurements; microbiological and chemical analyses) on raw materials, packaging components, in-process materials, finished goods, stability, retain, complaint or validation samples is chosen.

A service level agreement or contract must exist between the third-party lab and the client.

Some of the major benefits of third-party testing to the pharmaceutical industries could be

- Saves money and rework time by reducing the number of errors in the first place

YOUR COMPANY NAME

Name: _____ ID No.: _____ Issued by: _____

Designation: _____ Department: _____ Date: _____

- Reduces the workload of client lab
- Missing, ambiguous, unclear issues are identified and rectified in the early development stages of the product
- Reduces the number of defects released into production
- Verifies that the technical design conforms to the requirements and expectations of the user

GENERAL

1. The laboratory must establish a system like a contract, purchase order or SOP which clearly defines the responsibilities (including documentation) of both parties.
2. The document should also specify the person responsible for data review of the third party.
3. The customer lab must provide periodic audit of the third-party laboratories through an established mechanism.
4. Customers' laboratory must also verify accreditation of third party by an independent accreditation body.
5. In case a health regulatory body or GMP authority also audits the third party, the audit report must be available for the customer lab review when needed. Under such circumstances, the customer laboratory should verify corrective measures taken as a result of inspections.
6. Ensure adequate instructions provided to the third-party lab for testing of products.
7. Contract must be clearly written and documented regarding the use of quality standard methods as to which method will be used.
8. If the customer's lab test methods are intended for testing, then system must be in place to first carry out method transfer of those quality test methods.
9. For third-party testing, a system must be formulated to delineate data reporting from the third party to the customer's lab.
10. The written procedure should also define the responsibilities for data review as well as acceptance and rejection of those at the third-party lab.
11. Data trending must also be performed either at the third party or the customer lab. In either case, the procedure should be clearly outlined in the written procedure.

QCT-01.12

Good Documentation Practices

YOUR COMPANY NAME

Name: _____ ID No.: _____ Issued by: _____

Designation: _____ Department: _____ Date: _____

DOCUMENTATION

Documentation is a system, which manages and controls all documents during various activities performed in a pharmaceutical organization. Regulatory auditors rely highly on what the documents tell them. If it is not documented, it has not been done. The purpose of good documentation practices is to clearly document the actions that took place in the development, manufacture, testing and releasing for commercial use of a drug, biologics, vaccine, medical device, and so on. Documentation is required to assure the safety, identity, strength, purity and quality of the drug product and incorporates the following issues: responsibility and authority (for access, review, change, approval, issuance); control of routing, circulation, distribution and retrieval; interrelationships and consistency between documents; filing, traceability, retention, destruction, back-up and security; and quality (accurate, thorough, concise and timely). A controlled record is considered a legal document, so the data needs to be clearly documented for legal and preservation purposes.

PROCEDURE

1. The QC laboratory must have a system in place in the form of an SOP for the management and control of laboratory documentation related to analytical functions.
2. The policies and procedures at the site must outline the requirements for generation, review, approval and control of documents defining the receiving of samples, assigning work to analysts, testing and releasing of products.
3. Documentation control requirements must include
   a. Review and approval of SOPs prior to use

YOUR COMPANY NAME

Name: _____ ID No.: _____ Issued by: _____

Designation: _____ Department: _____ Date: _____

    b. Removal of obsolete SOPs, STMs, products specifications and other documents from the point of use

    c. Authorization and approval of changes to documents mentioned above

    d. A master list to identify the current revision of documents

    e. A system for assigning and controlling effective dates to SOPs and STMs

    f. Distribution to locations where they are used

    g. Master document retention requirements, with traceability

4. The procedures should clearly define a system for location-specific SOPs and STMs, including format to be used, approvals required for each type of document, maintenance of master copies, distribution, retrieval and archiving of obsolete documents.

5. The procedure for distribution and control of documents within the QC lab must be defined in the SOP as to how the documents will be distributed and controlled. The procedure also needs to emphasize that all records be secure, available and easily retrievable throughout the retention period.

6. The following instructions for a good documentation practice should also be incorporated in the SOP:

    a. The data must be entered directly in the controlled record and not on a piece of scrap paper for the interim period.

    b. The accuracy and legibility of the entries must be taken care of.

    c. Document's dates should be in standardized format as specified in the SOP. Backdates must strictly be avoided.

    d. All blank fields must be stricken out or put N/A with analyst's initials and date.

    e. Use water-resistant blue or black ink so that it does not fade over a period of time.

    f. Do not use pencils or markers to record data in the notebook.

    g. Each page in the controlled notebook should be numbered chronologically.

    h. Adhere to the notebook, with clear adhesive tape all printouts related to analysis with initials and date.

    i. Never use ditto marks when entering repetitive data.

QCT-01.13
Change Control

YOUR COMPANY NAME

Name: _____ ID No.: _____ Issued by: _____

Designation: _____ Department: _____ Date: _____

Change control is a monitoring system of reviewing and analysing the effect of a change, and to determine the need for corrective action to ensure that system retains its validated status.

The intent is to determine the need for action that would ensure that the system retains its validated status.

Change control in pharmaceutical industries is an important tool, which controls the change by

1. Identifying ownership of proposed change by qualified representative of appropriate discipline
2. Review and approval of proposed change
3. Preventing changes that could adversely affect product quality or conflict with registration or regulatory requirements
4. Assessing and monitoring the impact of the change

Changes may be needed for a variety of reasons, for example, new or improved functions, errors not detected earlier, alterations to accept new equipment in the system, updating the technical documents as per current compendial references, and so on. According to the procedure, actions are taken if a change is proposed to existing analytical equipment, STM, products specifications, starting material, product components, process equipment, process environment (or site), method of production or testing or any other change that may effect product quality or reproducibility of the process, to ensure the appropriate level of review, impact analysis and approval before making any change in the approved systems and ensures that sufficient supporting data are generated to demonstrate that the revised process will result in a product of the desired quality, consistent with the approved specifications.

YOUR COMPANY NAME

Name: _____ ID No.: _____ Issued by: _____

Designation: _____ Department: _____ Date: _____

UNPLANNED CHANGES

Unplanned changes are actually deviations and should be addressed using deviation handling procedures/non-conformance reporting system. Examples are as follows:

    a. Changes to processes
    b. Changes to design
    c. Changes to equipment and automated systems
    d. Changes to batch records, manufacturing instructions, SOPs
    e. Changes to analytical methods, specifications, raw materials

PLANNED CHANGES

Planned changes are intentional and pre-approved and can be permanent or temporary.

ROUTINE CHANGES (DOCUMENTATION)

1. The QC laboratory must initiate a procedure according to which the changes in the documents may be controlled.
2. The change control procedure must outline the types and categories of the documents and processes, which are governed by the change control SOP. According to the procedure, changes may involve the following technical documents on routine basis:
   a. STMs
   b. Standard control procedure
   c. Raw material specifications
   d. Finished product specifications
   e. Packaging material specifications
   f. SOPs
   g. Stability document
   h. Analytical instruments
3. Each document changed bears a revision number and the reason for revision, whereas the final document is reviewed and approved by QA unit.
4. The record will be maintained against the document number and revision number for each document and will include the following:
   a. Proposed changes
   b. Reason and justification for the changes proposed

YOUR COMPANY NAME

Name: _____ ID No.: _____ Issued by: _____

Designation: _____ Department: _____ Date: _____

    c. Impact of the change (validation/qualification requirement if changes are carried out)

    d. Notification of changes, regulatory aspect consideration

    e. Close-out

5. As per the procedure, any person of the lab can initiate the change request form unless otherwise instructed. The change initiating departmental head must, however, classify the change as minor, major and/or critical.

6. The change control form (CCF) will then be initiated with all the details including the current system, proposed change, reasons/justification and results to be accomplished, documents-related information and signed by the manager of the laboratory.

7. The change request form will be forwarded to the concerned documentation control department for assigning sequential number for traceability purpose and logbook entry. The documentation control department in the register marked "change control request" will maintain all the related details and sequential numbering.

8. The numbered CCF must then be returned back to the initiator review and impact analysis. The procedure must also outline the need of sending the CCF to other departments or sections, if needed, for their review and impact analysis.

9. The copies of the approved CCF will be forwarded to department concerned for making change and information (notification of change) to all directors.

10. The planned close-out date will be placed on the original CCF by the initiator in consultation with all departments affected by change and on the basis of the requirement to be fulfilled to formalize the change (as a result of review and impact analysis). Date of follow-up will also be specified.

11. The close-out date will be placed on the original CCF by the initiator when the changes have been formalized in the documents approved and the qualification/validation or any other requirement is completed.

12. The initiator department will forward the completed CCF with all the supporting drawing/documentations to the QA manager for review who will sign for the closeout and the completed CCF will be filed with the documentation control department.

QCT-02

Analytical Methods, Techniques and Quality Measures for Biological Products

QCT-02.1

Immunoblotting

YOUR COMPANY NAME

Name: _____ ID No.: _____ Issued by: _____

Designation: _____ Department: _____ Date: _____

The immunoblotting is an analytical technique used to detect specific proteins in a given sample of tissue homogenate or extract. It is a powerful and sensitive technique, which relies on the identification of single protein spots via antigen–antibody-specific reactions from 2D polyacrylamide gel electrophoresis (PAGE).

Proteins are typically separated by gel electrophoresis by the length of the polypeptide structure and transferred onto nitrocellulose membranes where they are detected using antibodies specific target proteins.

IMMUNOBLOTTING ANALYTICAL TECHNIQUE

1. In this technique, the membranes are first blocked with reagents to prevent non-specific binding of antibodies.
2. The primary antibodies, which recognize specific proteins, are then allowed to bind to their targets.
3. After the non-specific bindings are removed, secondary antibodies, which recognize the primary antibodies and have detection tags on them, are used.
4. After final washes, the detection tags, and thus indirectly the primary antibodies, are detected.
5. Detection tags on secondary antibodies are usually enzymes such as horseradish peroxidase (HRP) or alkaline phosphatase.
6. The probed membranes are treated with chemicals which react with the enzymes leading to the generation of light. This phenomenon is known as "chemiluminescence."
7. Immunoblotting is a good technique to detect proteins even if very small quantities of sample are available. It can detect as little as picogram amounts of protein, depending on the specificity of the antibodies.
8. Some of the disadvantages associated with this technique are
   a. It is a slow process and can detect only a few proteins per gel per day.
   b. Requires monoclonal or polyclonal antibodies which may be expensive to obtain commercially.

YOUR COMPANY NAME

Name: _____ ID No.: _____ Issued by: _____

Designation: _____ Department: _____ Date: _____

PROCEDURE

The immunoblotting is carried out in the following steps:

1. *Preparation of cell lysates*
   a. Harvest 70–85% confluent cells by trypsinization and spin.
   b. Lyse the pellet with 100 μL lysis buffer on ice for 10 min. If required, sample can be sonicated for not more than 5–10 s. The amount of lysis buffer depends on the number of cells available.
   c. Spin at 14,000 rpm (16,000 g) in an Eppendorf microfuge for 20 min at 4°C.
   d. Transfer the supernatant to a new tube and discard the pellet.
   e. Measure the protein concentration with protein assay.
   f. Mix equal amount of protein lysate from each sample separately with sample loading buffer and boil for 5 min. The final concentration of loading buffer must be 1×.
   g. Cool at room temperature (RT) for 5 min.
   h. Briefly spin to bring down the sample and loading buffer mixture prior to loading gel.

2. *Polyacrylamide gel*
   a. *Agarose plug:* 1% agarose dissolved in 1 × resolving gel buffer. (50 mL is made by melting it as needed, and re-adding water to maintain agarose conc.)
   b. *Resolving gel:* 24 mL of a 9% gel 5.4 mL 40% acrylamide/bisacrylamide (29:1 mix) 3 mL 8 × resolving gel buffer 15.6 mL water 12 μL tetramethylethylenediamine (TEMED) 60 μL 20% ammonium persulphate.
   c. *Stacking gel:* 8 mL 1 mL 40% acrylamide/bisacrylamide (29:1 mix) 2 mL 4 × stacking gel buffer 5 mL water 8 μL TEMED 21.6 μL 20% ammonium persulphate.

3. *Preparation of gel*
   a. Assemble the glass plates and spacers (1.5 mm thick).
   b. Pour an agarose plug (1–2 mm), which is prepared by dissolving 1% agarose in 1 × resolving gel buffer.
   c. Now add approximately 20 mL of running gel to about 1 cm below the wells of the comb and seal with 1 mL water-saturated 1-butanol.
   d. Pour off the butanol when gel has set and rinse with deionized water.
   e. Pour approximately 5 mL stacking gel and insert the comb immediately.

YOUR COMPANY NAME

Name: _____ ID No.: _____ Issued by: _____

Designation: _____ Department: _____ Date: _____

    f. When the stacking gel has set, place in gel rig and immerse in buffer.

    g. Flush the wells out thoroughly with running buffer before running the gel.

4. *Running the gel*
   a. The samples are loaded into the wells after brief spinning.
   b. Be sure to use protein markers.
   c. Run the gel with constant current of 100 V for about 1.5–2.5 h. Adjust the current later on according to the shift of bands.

5. *Preparation of membrane*
   a. Cut a piece of polyvinylidene difluoride (PVDF) membrane and wet it for about 30 min in methanol at RT.
   b. Remove methanol and add 1 × blotting buffer until ready to use.

6. *Membrane transfer*
   a. Assemble "sandwich" using a transfer.
   b. Pre-wet the sponges, filter papers (slightly bigger than gel) in 1 × blotting buffer.
      Sponge–filter paper–gel–membrane–filter paper–sponge
   c. Transfer for 1h at 1 amp constant current (or 100 V constant voltages) at 4°C on a stir plate. Bigger proteins might take longer time to transfer.
      Note: The time or current (or voltage) is different between laboratories. You can change them according to the apparatus you are using and your experience at the laboratory.
   d. When finished, immerse membrane in blocking buffer and block at 4°C overnight, or one hour at RT.
      Note: In order to get a good blot, it is suggested making the transferring buffer freshly every time a Western blotting is carried out.

7. *Antibodies and detection*
   a. Incubate with primary antibody diluted in Blocking buffer (usually, 5% milk) for 60 min at RT, or overnight at 4°C.
   b. Wash 3 × 5 min with 0.1% Tween 20 in phosphate buffered saline (PBS) (tris-buffered saline Tween-20 [TBST]).
   c. Incubate with secondary antibody diluted in blocking buffer for one hour at RT.
   d. Wash 3 × 10 min (or 4 × 5 min) with TBST.
   e. Detect with enhanced chemiluminescence (ECL).
      Note: If you want to look into both non-phosphor- and phosphor-protein with the same blot, make sure to probe the phosphor-antigen

YOUR COMPANY NAME

Name: _____ ID No.: _____ Issued by: _____

Designation: _____ Department: _____ Date: _____

first, and then to add proper phosphatase inhibitor during the Western blotting procedure due to the high activity of phosphatase. One would usually use phosphatase inhibitor cocktail and 50 mM sodium fluoride.

ENHANCED CHEMILUMINESCENCE

Chemiluminescence is the generation of electromagnetic radiation as light by the release of energy from a chemical reaction.

There are three types of chemiluminescent reactions:

1. Chemical reactions using synthetic compounds and usually involving a highly oxidized species such as peroxides are commonly termed chemiluminescent reactions.
2. Light-emitting reactions arising from a living organism, such as the firefly or jellyfish, are commonly termed bioluminescent reactions.
3. Light-emitting reactions which take place by the use of electrical current are designated electrochemiluminescent reactions.

The technique used for immunodetection protein identification is called ECL. It is a common technique for a variety of detection assays in biology.

With this technique proteins can be detected down to femtomole quantities, which is well below the detection limit for most assay systems.

1. Chemiluminescent detection methods depend on incubation of the Western blot with a substrate that will luminesce when exposed to the reporter on the secondary antibody.
2. In this technique, the PVDF membranes are first stained to visualize proteins, after which the immunodetection is undertaken. This allows matching of proteins detected with ECL against those detected with the non-specific protein stain through computer comparison of both images.
3. Chemiluminescent substrates for HRP are two-component systems consisting of a stable peroxide solution and an enhanced luminol solution.
4. To make a working solution, equal volumes of the two components are mixed together. The HRP enzyme is joined to the molecule of interest to form an enzyme complex. This is done through labelling an immunoglobulin that specifically recognizes the molecule.

YOUR COMPANY NAME

Name: _____ ID No.: _____ Issued by: _____

Designation: _____ Department: _____ Date: _____

5. The enhanced chemiluminescent substrate is converted into a sensitized reagent in the vicinity of the molecule of interest when incubated. This conversion is catalysed by the HRP-molecule enzyme complex.
6. A chemical reaction then occurs which produces light that can be detected by film or sensitive camera. During the reaction, the substrate produces a triplet carbonyl upon further oxidation by hydrogen peroxide, which emits light when it decays to the singlet carbonyl.
7. The image is analysed by densitometry, which evaluates the relative amount of protein staining and quantifies the results in terms of optical density.
8. The chemiluminescence procedure is carried out in a rotating oven at RT.

QCT-02.2

Gel Permeation Chromatography

YOUR COMPANY NAME

Name: _____ ID No.: _____ Issued by: _____

Designation: _____ Department: _____ Date: _____

Gel permeation chromatography (GPC), also known as size-exclusion chromatography (SEC) or gel filtration, is a widely accepted analytical method used in the separation, purification and characterization of biopolymers and synthetic polymers. GPC is a separation technique that involves transport of a liquid mobile phase through a column containing a porous material as the separation medium. The separation is based on differences in molecular size in solution. It is of particular importance for research in biological systems and has become by far the most widely used method for determining molecular weight distribution of synthetic polymers. Currently, most GPC analyses are performed by comparing the molecular weight of a sample against standards of known molecular weight. This method is often described as classical GPC.

BASIC PHILOSOPHY

1. The technique of GPC differs from other separation techniques such that it is based on the size or hydrodynamic volume of the analytes and utilizes a non-interactive mode of separation, whereas other separation techniques depend upon chemical or physical interactions to separate analytes.
2. The GPC employs a stationary phase composed of a macromolecular gel containing a porous network and hence affords a rapid method for the separation of oligomeric and polymeric species.
3. Separation occurs via the use of porous beads of glass or silica or a cross-linked gel packed in a column.
4. Specific columns are used for a range of different molecular weights that can be separated in them. Columns are steel cylinder typically 10 mm in diameter and 500–1000 mm in length.
5. When columns are created they are packed with porous beads with a specific pore size so that they are most accurate at separating molecules with sizes similar to the pore size.

YOUR COMPANY NAME

Name: _____ ID No.: _____ Issued by: _____

Designation: _____ Department: _____ Date: _____

6. It is worthwhile to note that a limited range of molecular weights can be separated by each column. Therefore, the size of the pores for the packing should be chosen as per the range of molecular weight of analytes that need to be separated.

7. The liquid mobile phase is usually water or a buffer for biological separations mixed with an organic solvent.

8. The solvent must first be assessed to be compatible with the column packing for synthetic polymer characterization.

9. The separation works on the strategy that the smaller analytes enter the pores more easily and spend more time in these pores, consequently increasing their retention time. On the other hand, the larger analytes spend relatively less time in the pores and are eluted quickly. In other words, molecules are separated by whether or not they can fit within the pore size of the packing material.

10. This phenomenon can be further understood in the following lines. Analytes are either retained completely or not retained at all depending on their size. As a molecule flows through the column, it passes through a number of porous beads. The force of diffusion draws in the molecules, which fit inside the pores. These molecules stay for a short while and then move on. If a molecule cannot fit into a pore, then it continues following the solvent flow.

11. The molecules that do not fit into the pores due to very small size of the pores will be eluted with the free volume of the particles (Vo). On the other hand, the analytes which are retained completely are eluted with the volume of solvent held in the pores (Vi). The following equation can determine the total volume (Vt), where Vg is the volume of the polymer gel; $Vt = Vg + Vi + Vo$.

12. The desired flow rate through the column can be achieved either by gravity or by using a high-pressure pump.

13. Careful selection of mobile phase and columns can optimize the SEC separation.

14. To separate hydrophilic samples, polar phases are best choice whereas for hydrophobic, non-polar phases work most effectively.

15. In order to design an effective SEC separation following parameters must be taken care of
    a. The interaction between sample and columns
    b. Mobile phase
    c. Size range of the pores
    d. Separating power or resolution

YOUR COMPANY NAME

Name: _____ ID No.: _____ Issued by: _____

Designation: _____ Department: _____ Date: _____

MECHANISM OF GEL PERMEATION CHROMATOGRAPHY

1. Like other types of chromatographic techniques (HPLC, GC), in GPC also, samples of interest are injected at the head of the column.
2. While travelling through the column, the small-sized molecules enter all pores larger than their size. Whereas the larger molecules have relatively less number of pores available for them to fit in since there will be less pores available larger than the size of these molecules.
3. Therefore the amount of pore volume available for larger molecules will be less than those for the small-sized molecules. Hence, the larger-sized molecules will elute faster.
4. In this way the sample emerges from the column in the inverse order of molecular size, which means that the largest molecule will elute first followed by progressively smaller molecules.
5. A concentration detector is located at the end of the column to determine the amount of sample emerging out.

ADVANTAGES OF GPC

1. The GPC technique can provide narrow bands despite the fact that polymer samples have broad ranges of molecular weights present.
2. This technique allows quick and easy estimation of molecular weights and distribution of polymer samples.
3. Low chance of loss of analytes since they do not interact chemically or physically with the columns.
4. GPC provides a more convenient method of determining the molecular weights of polymers.
5. The separation time is well defined because there is a final elution volume for all non-retained analytes.
6. The total time duration for most samples does not exceed more than an hour.
7. GPC is often used as a quality control measure for polymer production. This includes both product release testing as well as product failure analysis.
8. Many of the most crucial properties of a polymer, for example, strength, elongation and crucial processing parameters, depend upon its molecular weight. Therefore, molecular weight determination is a good way to predict a polymer's behaviour. Classical GPC analysis plays an important role in serving this function.

YOUR COMPANY NAME

Name: _____ ID No.: _____ Issued by: _____

Designation: _____ Department: _____ Date: _____

9. Multidetector GPC is often the best choice for high-end applications such as drug delivery polymers. These systems tend to be more complex and include a more unique polymer architecture.

DISADVANTAGES

1. The limited number of peaks that can be resolved within the short timescale of the run is one of the disadvantages of GPC.

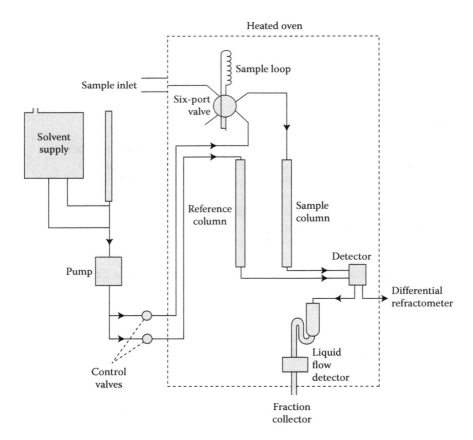

FIGURE 2.1   Gel permeation chromatograph.

YOUR COMPANY NAME

Name: _____ ID No.: _____ Issued by: _____

Designation: _____ Department: _____ Date: _____

2. Another disadvantage of GPC for polymers is that a filtration has to be done before using the instrument so that the dust and particulates may not destroy columns.
3. Presence of dust or other particulates may also interfere with the detectors. This again necessitates the filtration before using the instrument.
4. The pre-filtration, although useful and necessary, may remove higher molecular weight samples before loading on the column.

Figure 2.1 shows diagrammatic presentation of gel permeation chromatograph.

QCT-02.3

Electrophoresis

YOUR COMPANY NAME

Name: _____ ID No.: _____ Issued by: _____

Designation: _____ Department: _____ Date: _____

The electrokinetic motion of dispersed particles relative to a fluid under the influence of a spatially uniform electric field is known as electrophoresis. Electrophoresis is a technique used in genetic testing to analyse and separate proteins, DNA and RNA.

Electrophoresis uses an electrical current to separate the molecules by electrical charge. This phenomenon works regardless of the physical arrangements for the apparatus, and the medium through which molecules are allowed to migrate. The method is based on the changes in the electrophoretic pattern of macromolecules through biospecific interaction or complex formation. The interaction of a charged or uncharged molecule normally changes its electrophoretic properties.

The analytical methods generally used in biotechnology laboratory are called affinity electrophoresis. This technique is useful in obtaining both qualitative and quantitative information. Affinity electrophoresis includes the mobility shift, the charge shift and the capillary electrophoresis.

The most common types of electrophoresis are

1. Gel electrophoresis
2. Capillary zone electrophoresis

GEL ELECTROPHORESIS

1. Gel electrophoresis separates the molecules by molecular weight and charge using different types of gel mediums that vary by the molecule being analysed.
2. The separation of molecules within a gel is determined by the relative size of the pores formed within the gel.
3. Many substances including starch gels and paper have served as media for electrophoresis. However, the most commonly used mediums for proteins; DNA and RNA separation are agarose and polyacrylamide.
4. The phenomenon of separation by molecular weight could be understood such that the gel is a cross-linked polymer whose composition and

YOUR COMPANY NAME

Name: _____ ID No.: _____ Issued by: _____

Designation: _____ Department: _____ Date: _____

porosity is selected on the basis of the specific weight and composition of the target to be analysed. The pore size of a gel is therefore determined by two factors:

    a. The total amount of acrylamide

    b. The amount of cross-linker

5. The gel composition for proteins with molecular weights ranging from 10,000 to 1,000,000 is 7½% acrylamide, whereas for higher molecular weight proteins, lower acrylamide gel concentrations are required.

6. As the total amount of acrylamide increases, the pore size decreases. If the molecule to be separated is protein or small nucleic acids (DNA, RNA or oligonucleotides) then the gel is composed of different concentrations of acrylamide and a cross-linker, producing different sized mesh networks of polyacrylamide.

7. For separation of larger nucleic acids greater than a few hundred bases, purified agarose is preferred.

8. The support medium for electrophoresis can be formed into a gel within a tube or it can be layered into flat sheets.

9. The tubes are used for one-dimensional (ID) separations, while the sheets have a larger surface area and are better for 2D separations.

10. Advantages of gel electrophoresis:

    a. The gel is easily poured and does not affect or denature the samples

    b. The samples can also be recovered

11. Disadvantages of gel electrophoresis:

    a. The electrophoresis process can melt the gels

    b. The buffer can become exhausted

    c. Different forms of genetic material may run in unpredictable forms

12. The gel electrophoresis can further be categorized into three types:

    a. DNA electrophoresis

    b. One-dimensional electrophoresis or ID

    c. Two-dimensional electrophoresis or 2D

DNA ELECTROPHORESIS

a. This technique is used to separate DNA fragments by size. In this type of electrophoresis, agarose gel is used for the separation of large DNA molecules, whereas polyacrylamide is a better choice for short DNA fragments.

YOUR COMPANY NAME

Name: _____ ID No.: _____ Issued by: _____

Designation: _____ Department: _____ Date: _____

b. The agarose gels are submerged in buffer used for the separation, typically tris-borate-EDTA (TBE) or tris-acetate-EDTA (TAE), that is why the technique is also known as submarine electrophoresis.

c. Among a number of buffers used for agarose gel electrophoresis, TAE, TBE and sodium borate (SB) are the most commonly used ones.

d. TAE has the lowest buffering capacity but provides the best resolution for larger DNA. The smaller fragments of DNA move faster through the gel matrix and larger fragments move slower. The gel can be made so that its pores are just the right.

e. Dimensions for separating molecules within a specific range of sizes and shapes. Smaller fragments usually travel further than large ones. Following the separation, the gels can be stained or transferred.

f. The equipment and supplies necessary for conducting DNA electrophoresis are relatively simple and include
- An electrophoresis chamber and power supply
- Gel casting trays. The open ends of the trays are closed with tape while the gel is being cast, then removed prior to electrophoresis
- Sample combs around which molten agarose is poured to form sample wells in the gel
- Electrophoresis buffer
- Loading buffer, which contains a dense material like glycerol to allow the sample to "fall" into the sample wells, and one or two tracking dyes, which migrate in the gel and allow visual monitoring or how far the electrophoresis has proceeded
- Ethidium bromide, a fluorescent dye used for staining nucleic acids
- Transilluminator, used to visualize ethidium bromide-stained DNA in gels

g. The separated DNA is then detected by dyes that bind to the molecules and are viewed under UV illumination.

h. Capillary or electrical transfer for probing can transfer the nucleic acids from the gel matrix to membrane sheets.

ONE-DIMENSIONAL (1D) ELECTROPHORESIS

a. This type of electrophoresis is a simple, rapid and sensitive analytical tool used to separate protein molecules and nucleic acids based on physical characteristics such as size, shape or isoelectric point.

b. The technique is also known as PAGE.

YOUR COMPANY NAME

Name: _____ ID No.: _____ Issued by: _____

Designation: _____ Department: _____ Date: _____

    c. Most systems for protein separation are designed in a vertical format, which allows for air to be excluded during casting. Gels are then either suspended between or submerged into buffer tanks for separation.

    d. For 1D protein gels, combs are used to form wells in which liquid samples can be applied. An electrical field is passed through the medium containing the target mixture to allow proteins to migrate.

    e. The travelling rate for each type of molecule through the medium varies according to its electrical charge or size.

    f. Following the separation, the gels can be stained by chromagenic stains or by fluorescent stains in order to detect the proteins.

TWO-DIMENSIONAL (2D) ELECTROPHORESIS

    a. The 2D electrophoresis begins with 2D electrophoresis but then separates the molecules by a second property in a direction of 90° from the first.

    b. When the proteins are separated in one dimension, all the molecules lie along a lane but be separated from each other by a property called isoelectric point or the pH at which at which the molecule carries no electrical charge.

    c. The result is that the molecules are spread uniformly across a 2D gel.

    d. Two-dimensional electrophoresis is a more effective technique than 1D electrophoresis because it is unlikely that two molecules will be similar in two distinct properties. Therefore, molecules are more effectively separated in 2D electrophoresis compared to 1D electrophoresis.

CAPILLARY ELECTROPHORESIS

    1. Capillary electrophoresis (CE) offers many advantages for the separation of a wide variety of molecules.

    2. CE encompasses a family of related separation techniques that use narrow-bore fused-silica capillaries to separate ionic species based on their size to charge ratio in the interior of a small capillary filled with an electrolyte (see Figure 2.2).

    3. The separations are made possible by the use of high voltages.

    4. The CE system comprises of the following components:

        a.   Sample vial

        b.   Source and destinations vials

        c.   Capillary

        d.   Electrodes

YOUR COMPANY NAME

Name: _____ ID No.: _____ Issued by: _____

Designation: _____ Department: _____ Date: _____

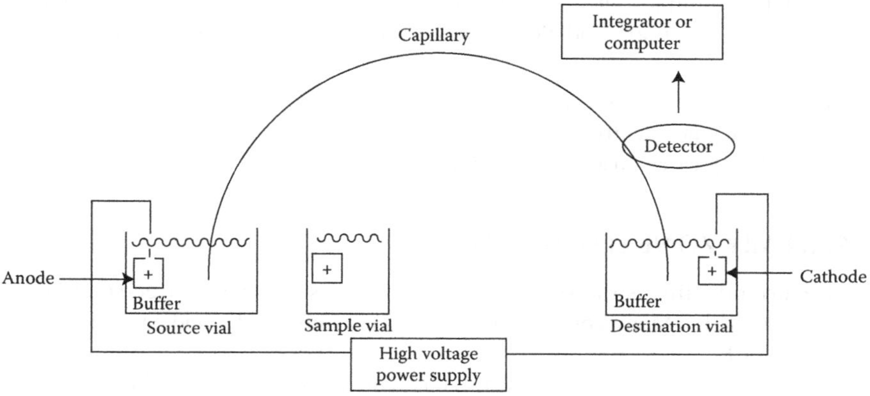

FIGURE 2.2 Diagrammatic presentation of capillary electrophoresis system.

   e. High-voltage power supply
   f. Detector
   g. Data output and handling device
5. Sample introduction is accomplished by immersing the end of the capillary into a sample vial and applying pressure, vacuum or voltage.
6. The applied electric field between the source and destination vials initiates the migration of analytes.
7. The velocity of migration of an analyte in CE depends up on the rate of electro-osmotic flow (EOF) of the buffer solution.
8. The EOF helps to pull the negative and positive ions through the capillary.
9. During the migration phase, separation of electrolytes takes place according to their electrophoretic mobility.
10. Typically the EOF is directed towards the negatively charged cathode so that the buffer flows through the capillary from the source vial to the destination vial. It is also because the EOF of the buffer solution is generally greater than that of the EOF of the analytes; all analytes are carried along with the buffer solution towards the cathode.
11. These analytes are then detected at the outlet end of capillary. The output of the detector is sent to a data handling device or integrator, which displays the data as an electropherogram.
12. Peaks at different retention times in the electropherogram demonstrate the separation of chemical compounds.

YOUR COMPANY NAME

Name: ————————— ID No.: ——————— Issued by: ————

Designation: ————— Department: ————— Date: —————

The CE technique can further be sub-categorized into different types, based on the types of capillary and electrolytes used. These categories include

   a. Capillary zone electrophoresis (CZE)
   b. Capillary gel electrophoresis (CGE)
   c. Capillary isoelectric focusing (CIEF)

CAPILLARY ZONE ELECTROPHORESIS

   1. Currently, this is the simplest form of CE, also known as free-solution CE (FSCE). Many compounds can be separated rapidly and easily using the CZE.
   2. In this technique, the separation mechanism is based on differences in the electrophoretic mobilities of the analytes resulting in different velocities of migration of ionic species in the electrophoretic buffer contained in the capillary.
   3. Fundamental to CZE are homogeneity of the buffer solution and constant field strength throughout the length of the capillary.
   4. The separation relies principally on the pH-controlled dissociation of acidic groups on the solute or the protonation of basic functions on the solute.

CAPILLARY GEL ELECTROPHORESIS

   1. CGE is the adaptation of traditional gel electrophoresis into the capillary using polymers in solution to create a molecular sieve also known as replaceable physical gel.
   2. This allows analytes having similar charge-to-mass ratios to be resolved by size. This technique is commonly employed in SDS-gel molecular weight analysis of proteins and the sizing of applications of DNA sequencing and genotyping.
   3. This is a high-resolution alternative to slab gel electrophoresis.

CAPILLARY ISOELECTRIC FOCUSING

   1. Isoelectric focusing is a type of zone electrophoresis for separating different molecules by their electric charge differences.

YOUR COMPANY NAME

Name: _____ ID No.: _____ Issued by: _____

Designation: _____ Department: _____ Date: _____

2. It takes advantage of the fact that a molecule's charge changes with the pH of its surroundings. It allows amphoteric molecules, such as proteins, to be separated in a pH gradient generated between the cathode and anode.

3. Proteins show considerable variation in iso-electric points, but pI values usually fall in the range of 3–12 pH, whereas majority of them having pIs between pH 4 and pH 7.

4. A protein that is in a pH region below its isoelectric point (pI) will be positively charged and will migrate towards the cathode. The ones being in pH region above their pI values will carry a negative charge and will move towards anode.

5. As the positive charged molecule migrates through a gradient of decreasing pH, the protein's overall charge will decrease by either loosing or gaining an electron. This results in slowing down the migration until the protein reaches the pH region that corresponds to its pI.

6. At the solutes isoelectric point (pI), it has no net charge and migration stops and the sample is focused into a tight zone.

7. In CIEF, once a solute has focused at its pI, with each protein positioned at a point in the pH gradient to its pI, the proteins condense into sharp bands in the pH gradient at their individual characteristic pI values.

QCT-02.4

Ion-Exchange Chromatography

YOUR COMPANY NAME

Name: _____ ID No.: _____ Issued by: _____

Designation: _____ Department: _____ Date: _____

Ion-exchange chromatography (IEC) is a process that allows the separation of ions and polar molecules based on charge–charge interactions between the proteins in the sample. In biochemistry it is widely used to separate charged molecules. An important area of the application is extraction and purification of biologically produced substances such as proteins and amino acids, for example, DNA and RNA. IEC can also be used for the separation of peptides and oligonucleotides.

Ion-exchange resin consists of an insoluble matrix with charge groups covalently attached. The charged groups are associated with mobile counterions, which can be reversibly exchanged with other ions of the same charge without altering the matrix. To optimize binding of all charged molecules, the mobile phase is generally a low-to-medium conductivity (salt concentration) solution. Ion-exchange separations are carried out in a column, by a batch procedure or by expanded bed adsorption.

The matrix may be based on inorganic compounds, synthetic resins or polysaccharides. The characteristics of the matrix determine its chromatographic properties such as efficiency, capacity and recovery as well as its chemical stability.

Exchangers could be both positively and negatively charged.

Based on the difference of charges, the technique is therefore subdivided into

a. Cation-exchange chromatography (CEC), where the positively charged ions bind to a negatively charged resin
b. Anion-exchange chromatography (AEC), in which the resins are positively charged and binding ions are negative

Figure 2.3 shown below could easily explain the above-mentioned phenomenon.

Figure 2.3a depicts a cation-exchange resin which has positive charged ions bound to it whereas in Figure 2.3b, positively charged resin has negative binding ions.

93

YOUR COMPANY NAME

Name: _____ ID No.: _____ Issued by: _____

Designation: _____ Department: _____ Date: _____

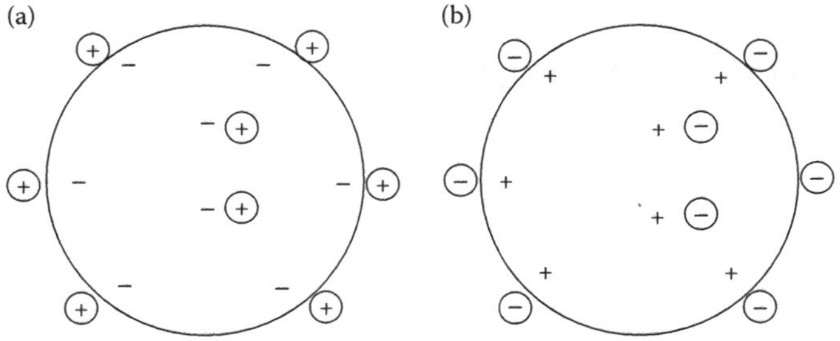

FIGURE 2.3 Diagrammatic presentation of cation- and anion-exchange chromatography.

The adsorption of the molecules to the solid support is driven by the ionic interaction between the two moieties and binding capacities are generally quite high.

1. The number and location of the charges on the molecule and solid support determine the strength of the interaction.
2. By increasing the salt concentration (generally a linear salt gradient) the molecules with the weakest ionic interactions are disrupted first and elute earlier in the salt gradient.
3. Those molecules that have a very strong ionic interaction require a higher salt concentration and elute later in the gradient.

EFFECT OF CHARGE ON THE PROTEIN MOLECULE

In the IEC, charge on the protein has significant effects on its behaviour. There are many ionizable groups present on the side chains of protein's amino acids as well as their amino- and carboxyl-termini. These include basic groups on the side chains of lysine, arginine and histidine and acidic groups on the side chains or glutamate, aspartate, cysteine and tyrosine. The charge on each side chain is influenced by the pH of the solution, the pK of the side chain and the side chain's environment. The relationship between pH, pK and charge for individual amino acids can be described by the Henderson–Hasselbalch equation:

$$pH = pK + \log\frac{[\text{conjugate base}]}{[\text{conjugate acid}]}$$

In general terms, as the pH of a solution increases, deprotonation of the acidic and basic groups on proteins occur, so that carboxyl groups are converted to

YOUR COMPANY NAME

Name: _____ ID No.: _____ Issued by: _____

Designation: _____ Department: _____ Date: _____

carboxylate anions (R-COOH to R-COO⁻) and ammonium groups are converted to amino groups ($R\text{-}NH_3^+$ to $R\text{-}NH_2$). In proteins the pI is defined as the pH at which a protein has no net charge. When the pH > pI, a protein has a net negative charge, and when the pH < pI, a protein has a net positive charge. The pI varies for different proteins.

PROTEIN SEPARATION BY IEC

1. Separation of proteins through IEC occurs according to their net charges which is dependent on the composition of the mobile phase.
2. There are numerous functional groups in the protein molecules that can have both positive and negative charges. By adjusting the pH of the mobile phase, various protein molecules can be separated.
3. The process of using the ion exchanger, in protein or enzyme purification goes like this:
   a. Equilibrate the cation exchanger with low salt concentration buffer of desired pH.
   b. Apply the enzyme in the same buffer at the same pH and salt concentration.
   c. Wash the unbound ions away using the equilibration buffer.
   d. An increase in the pH of the mobile phase buffer results in the decrease in positive charge of the molecule by becoming less protonated.
   e. This in turn decreases the capability of the molecule to form a strong ionic interaction with the negatively charged solid support and hence causes the molecule to elute from the chromatography column.
4. This could be further understood by another example; if a protein has a net positive charge at pH 7, then it will bind to a column of negatively charged beads, whereas a negatively charged protein would not. By changing the pH so that the net charge on the protein is negative, it will also be eluted.

There are two basic types of ion exchangers: those for binding positively charged ions or cations, which display on their surface negatively charged groups; and those for binding negatively charged ions or anions, which display on their surface positively charged groups.

The ion exchanger is composed of the solid support material, which for enzymes and proteins must be a "hydrogel" or polymer composed for easily hydrated groups like cellulose consisting of polymers of sugar molecules. On the

YOUR COMPANY NAME

Name: _____ ID No.: _____ Issued by: _____

Designation: _____ Department: _____ Date: _____

surface of the polymeric support material, ionic groups are displayed which have been covalently linked to the polymer support. Here are models of ion exchangers:

ANION-EXCHANGE CHROMATOGRAPHY

This analytical technique is practiced with either a strong or a weak anion exchange column, containing a quaternary ammonium ion, or with a weak anion exchanger, having either a tertiary or secondary amine functional group, such as diethylaminoethyl group.

ANION EXCHANGERS FUNCTIONAL GROUP

Diethylaminoethyl (DEAE) -O-CH_2-CH_2-N+H (CH_2CH_3)$_2$
Quaternary aminoethyl (QAE) -O-CH_2-CH_2-N+(C_2H_5) 2-CH_2-CHOH-CH_3
Quaternary ammonium (Q) -O-CH_2-CHOH-CH_2-O-CH_2-CHOH-CH_2-N+ (CH_3)$_3$

1. The high capacity and ability of the matrixes in AEC to bind up and separate fragmented nucleic acids and lipopolysaccharides from the initial slurry, makes it a primary chromatography step. Matrixes have capacity to bind from 10 to 100 mg of protein per mL.
2. Typically, AEC is performed using buffers at pH between 7 and 10 and running a gradient from a solution containing just this buffer to a solution containing this buffer with 1M NaCl.
3. The salt in the solution competes for binding to the immobilized matrix and releases the protein from its bound state at a given concentration.
4. Proteins separate because the amount of salt needed to compete varies with the external charge of the protein.
5. Uses of AEC include initial clean-up of crude slurry, separation of proteins from each other, concentrating a protein, and the removal of negatively charged endotoxin from protein preparations.

CATION-EXCHANGE CHROMATOGRAPHY

This technique of separation is less commonly used compared to anion exchange. The main reason behind this is the fact that often proteins do not stick to this resin at physiological pHs and one is reluctant to titrate a protein through its isoelectric

YOUR COMPANY NAME

Name: _____ ID No.: _____ Issued by: _____

Designation: _____ Department: _____ Date: _____

point to get it to adhere to the resin. However, the technique is equally prevailing as AEC for initial separations with equivalently high capacity.

1. Characteristically, CEC is performed with buffers at pHs between 4 and 7.
2. The CEC is run on gradient from a solution containing the buffer only to a solution containing the buffer with 1 M NaCl.
3. CEC use includes
   a. Initial clean-up of a crude slurry
   b. Separation of proteins from each other
   c. Concentrating a protein

   As a common first purification step for proteins expressed under acidic conditions such as in *P. pastoris*

CATION EXCHANGERS FUNCTIONAL GROUP

Carboxymethyl (CM) -O-CH$_2$-COO
Sulphopropyl (SP) -O-CH$_2$-CHOH-CH$_2$-O-CH$_2$-CH$_2$-CH$_2$SO$_3$
Methyl sulphonate (S) -O-CH$_2$-CHOH-CH$_2$-O-CH$_2$-CHOH-CH$_2$SO$_3$
Sulphonic and quaternary amino groups are used to form strong ion exchangers.

QCT-03
Laboratory Training Manual

QCT-03.1

Laboratory Safety and Good Laboratory Practice

YOUR COMPANY NAME

Name: _____ ID No.: _____ Issued by: _____

Designation: _____ Department: _____ Date: _____

Provide training to the QC staff (especially new staff) regarding laboratory safety and GLPs.

PROCEDURE

1. The QC manager is responsible to maintain separate training log for the analyst.
2. Good housekeeping and safety: Walk around the laboratory showing items of importance such as fire exits, fire extinguishers, storage area and the different types of waste bins. Mention the cost of some of the high technology equipment and explain the importance of proper care of such items. Explain bench layouts and the services provided to them, the fume cupboard, at this time mention about the hazards involved with compressed gases and vacuum equipment.

   Bring to the employees' attention, their responsibilities (under the health and duties of the company policy). Introduce the departmental safety & fire fighting representative and ask them to explain their duties and the working of the safety & fire fighting unit.

   2.1. *Personal hygiene and clothing.* Explain the need for cleanliness and the avoidance of contamination; this should include the location and use of the emergency shower and eyewash.

      Point out that whenever in the laboratory, working or not, safety spectacles and fastened laboratory coat should be worn. Explain the importance of washing hands before eating and drinking and why eating, drinking or applying cosmetics in the labs is hazardous, and that the aforementioned items plus smoking are forbidden.

   2.2. *Accidents and illness.* Explain where medical centre (clinic) is located and the position of the laboratory first-aid box. Run

YOUR COMPANY NAME

Name: _____ ID No.: _____ Issued by: _____

Designation: _____ Department: _____ Date: _____

through the steps to be taken in case of burns, both heat and chemical, bleeding, falls gassing and electrical shock (see section on building evacuation plan in case of any emergency). Make sure the new recruit is aware that all accidents, no matter how trivial, should be notified to the safety officer and departmental manager as soon as possible.

2.3. *Fire.* Cover the types of fire that may occur and the correct type of extinguisher to deal with. Show the new employees all the fire exits from the laboratory, the location of the fire alarms, the assembly point and make sure that the fire exit procedure and evacuation plan in case of emergency is read fully and understood.

2.4. *Chemical hazards.* Cover the ways in which chemicals can get into the body, that is, inhalation, ingestion, skin absorption and injection, and the appropriate steps to be taken to prevent the above happening. Emphasize the need to use safety carriers for carrying large bottles and flasks.

Point out the storage area for flammable chemicals, both the small cupboards with the laboratory, pointing out that no more than 50 litres may be held within the laboratory at any one time and preferably much less, and the main external solvent store. Explain the procedure within the laboratory with working flammable liquids so that no other member of staff uses a source of ignition; at this point restate that smoking is not permitted within the laboratory. Point out the compounds (containing ether linkages) may form peroxides, which present a fire and explosion hazard.

At this point make the following statements most frequently:

1. Never pipette by mouth (make sure that a pipette filler has been issued).
2. Never use chemicals for medicinal purposes and never taste the chemicals, unless specifically told to do so and only if all other tests are satisfactory.
3. Explain the correct use of fume cupboards and their limitations.
4. Show the position and use of the cyanide antidote.

2.5. *Waste disposal.* Explain the system for disposal of excess samples, that is, raw materials, tablets, and so on.

YOUR COMPANY NAME

Name: _____ ID No.: _____ Issued by: _____

Designation: _____ Department: _____ Date: _____

2.5.1. Explain that the disposal of chemical waste is dictated by its nature and toxicity. Whenever possible, toxic materials should be neutralized and detoxified; small amounts of certain materials may be flushed down the sink, in a fume cupboard if necessary, approved by a senior member of staff. Larger amounts must be correctly packed and labelled for the house-keeping department to arrange for disposal.

2.5.2. In the cases of flammable liquids which are water miscible and of low toxicity and small quantity, they may be flushed down a sink with a large amount of water, if the liquid is immiscible, either evaporate on a steam bath taking the normal precautions for flammable liquid work or in the case of halogenated types, use the solvent waste container.

2.6. *Emissions.* Explain the hazards of the UV lamp and proper use of the ultrasonic bath.

2.7. *Electrical equipment.* Do not try to repair equipment—hazards of low and high voltage. Report any obvious deterioration, for example, cables, and so on.

2.8. *Safe use of equipment.* Explain that glass joints should be lubricated to prevent sticking. Closed vessels should never be heated or cooled unless instructed to do so, and should be used only after taking suitable precautions. Demonstrate correct method of cutting glass tubing, and fitting glass tubing into corks and rubber bungs, give examples of the possible emphasis that glass and other "sharps" have their own special waste disposal systems that must be adhered to.

2.9. Never carry out an unauthorized experiment.

2.10. The above points relate to both chemical and microbiological laboratories. The points below are of importance to the trainee within the microbiological control laboratory.

2.10.1. All biological materials including blood and microorganisms must be regarded as hazardous and potential sources of infection.

2.10.2. Avoid at all costs direct contact with any organism. Any external part of the body, which comes into contact with biological material, should be thoroughly washed with disinfectant/ antiseptic solutions immediately, for example, Radol or Savlon 1% solution of Vikron from Antec International UK.

YOUR COMPANY NAME

Name: _____ ID No.: _____ Issued by: _____

Designation: _____ Department: _____ Date: _____

2.10.3. If ingestion of biological material occurs, the mouth should be thoroughly rinsed with water. It should be followed by medical aid, no matter how trivial it may seem.

2.10.4. In all cases, the laboratory supervisor, manager and safety officer should be informed and an accident form should be filled.

2.10.5. All the pipettes, microscope slides, inoculating loops, or any other equipment used for handling blood or microorganisms, must be sterilized immediately after use.

2.10.6. A pipette pot is allocated to each member of the laboratory staff and, as such it is their personal responsibility to change the disinfectant on a weekly basis.

2.10.7. On removal of pipettes from the pots, they are washed thoroughly and then re-sterilized at 100°C for 2 h. Only after this second sterilizing procedure, the pipettes can be put back into use.

2.10.8. Biological contaminated materials—all waste materials contaminated with microorganism, blood, and so on—must first of all be sterilized before being made available for collection by the cleaner.

Non-flammable materials must be totally immersed in strong disinfectant solution for at least half an hour. Flammables must be put in special autoclave bags, which are sealed and autoclaved at 15 psi for 30 min, before transfer to the company incinerator or a burning pit.

2.10.9. In the case of spillage, the affected area should be soaked in disinfectant for half an hour. Any glassware (picked up broken glass with forceps) must be sterilized at 180°C for 2 hours before being put back into normal use. Any clothes used to mop up spillage should be treated as in Section 2.10.8 (flammables). This applies to contaminated or potential contaminated rubber gloves as well.

GOOD LABORATORY PRACTICES

2.11. Importance of analytical work should be emphasized for

2.11.1. Ensuring safe products and upholding company's reputation

YOUR COMPANY NAME

Name: _____ ID No.: _____ Issued by: _____

Designation: _____ Department: _____ Date: _____

2.11.2. Detecting trace toxic impurities, identification, and so on

2.11.3. Respect of Medicine Act, Professional bodies, and so on

2.12. Explain the importance to follow approved methods and emphasize that no alternation or short cuts are to be made to the approved.

2.13. Explain how specification is derived from the BP, EP and USP.

2.14. State that, when in doubt, seek assistance from senior analysts only, and point that this seeking of assistance will be seen in a much better light than going down a blind alley on a speculative hunch.

2.15. Explain what SOPs are and the importance of following them.

2.16. Explain how different tests can have different degrees of accuracy—significant of result.

2.17. Explain the expiry date system used on certain reagents.

2.18. Show how a laboratory notebook should be laid out, including the fact that all figures should be directly entered in pen not pencil. All alternative (correction, if necessary) should be crossed out but left legible and initiated with an explanation, if required.

2.19. Explain the consequences of fiddling results—possible dismissal and prosecution.

2.20. Explain the importance of raw data storage, spectra, chromatograms, and so on and their correct labelling and cross-referencing.

2.21. Explain the limitations in some methods, for example, interference in iron limit test, and so on and what to look for, for example, limit of detection.

2.22. Explain the difference between accuracy and precision and how errors can be minimized.

2.23. Show areas where books for reference are kept within the laboratory.

2.24. Explain other sources of information, such as the files.
Explain once more that the trainee is being employed in a responsible position and, as such, is expected and required to perform his/her duties properly and diligently.

QCT-03.2

Training of Sampling Procedure

YOUR COMPANY NAME

Name: _____ ID No.: _____ Issued by: _____

Designation: _____ Department: _____ Date: _____

Provide training in accordance with a written program for the sampling.

PROCEDURE

1. Describe the importance of sampling.
2. The reliance of analytical results or sampling.
3. Explain the QA check on vendor improvement.
   3.1. Sampling is as important as analysis, for unless sampling is carried out satisfactorily no reliance can be placed on analytical results. Also, the sampler may be the only person in quality unit to see the bulk container and its contents. He is therefore in a position to report any abnormalities that may not be apparent in a laboratory examination of the samples taken. Wrongly taken or contaminated samples would almost certainly result in time being wasted in repeating analysis and could adversely affect the product or material data.
   3.2. *Submission of material for analysis.* Explain how incoming materials are booked-in and the flow of documentation and labelling. Indicate the information the sampler gets from the labels, material receiving report, containers and where the sampler signs to show the material has been sampled.
   3.3. *Avoidance of contamination.* Explain that great care should be taken to avoid contamination of both bulk material and samples. Clean equipment must be used for each material sampled and for the following container sampled if the previous sample is abnormal. Spatulas/scoops, and so on, must be cleaned after use by washing in hot, soapy water and rinsing thoroughly before drying with a clean fibre-free cotton cloth. If necessary, a suitable solvent, for example, 70% alcohol, may be used to remove water immiscible

YOUR COMPANY NAME

Name: _____ ID No.: _____ Issued by: _____

Designation: _____ Department: _____ Date: _____

material first. Pipettes should be similarly cleaned, rinsed with alcohol and finally blown dry with a gentle current of air.

Overalls should not be dirty unreasonably and hair-covering cap and face mask should be worn. Breast pockets should not be used for pens, and so on as objects could fall into containers. It is necessary to clean the outside of containers and liners before attempting to take samples. When drums are sampled "on-end," make sure that all dirt and water are removed from the recess around the closure. Spray liners with 70% alcohol. The sampler should arrange for any spillages to be cleaned up as soon as possible either by vacuum and or by hosing with water if unavoidable. To reduce the risk of contaminating samples required for microbiological analysis, they should always be taken before any others required.

3.4. *Labelling of containers and sampler.* Explain to the sampler that checking the labelling of bulk containers and correct labelling of samples is extremely important, particularly as product names can be very similar with little differences. Do not make labels in advance. Make them only before their usage, for example, manganous gluconate, magnesium gluconate.

The name should always be checked against code numbers, as given on sampling sheets, SOPs, specifications and material-receiving report.

The information on the containers should be the same as on documents. Containers of purchased good should, on receipt, bear the name of the material on the container or on label affixed to the container. The sampler should satisfy himself as far as possible that the supplier agrees with respect to the identity of material.

When in doubt, he should consult the laboratory responsible for testing the material. The sample labels should be affixed immediately to the bottles before filling.

Sample names/batch number should not be marked on bottle caps, as this can lead to confusion. Do not transfer the small quantities of samples to another product container of different identity (while dispensing).

3.5. *Suitability of bulk containers and storage conditions.* Explain that the sampler must report instances when material is packed in unsuitable or badly damaged containers or stored under unsuitable conditions. Contamination of the containers with other materials or the

YOUR COMPANY NAME

Name: ——————————— ID No.: ——————————— Issued by: ——————

Designation: ————————— Department: ————————— Date: ————————————

presence of foreign odours or dampness must be reported. The information and any others adverse comments on the contents of containers should be recorded on the submission document. Special consideration will be made only after testing and appropriate approvals by QA manager, QC manager and quality affairs director only.

3.6. *Sampling procedures*

    3.6.1. Show and explain the use of the following equipment to take samples:

        Spatula/scoop (stainless steel and nickel)

        Sampling spear

        Self adhesive tape

        Bottle carriers

        Sampling containers

        Amber glass (both powder and liquid and the appropriate cap/wads)

        Securitainers

        Polythene bottles

        Plastic bags

        Sterilized spatulas, bottles, and so on required for microbiological samples

    3.6.2. General procedure prior to sampling:

        Explain that before sampling a batch, the sampler consults the sampling SOP and determines the size and number of the samples to be taken by reference to the sampling instructions.

All materials for sampling must be moved to the appropriate sampling booth before being opened. The sampler then collects together the appropriate number and size of bottles.

Once the required number of bottles have been labelled and placed in carriers, the sampler ensures that he has sufficient spatulas, scoops, and so on to enable a clean tool to be used for each product to be sampled and then proceeds to the appropriate stores area.

Note 1: Training in the practicalities of sampling is best carried out using the "sitting with Nellie" technique, that is, the trainer initially demonstrates each procedure then ensures that the sampler can satisfactorily carry out the same technique.

Note 2: Cover the requirements of SOP relating to the sampling materials. Sampling should be performed under HEPA filters.

YOUR COMPANY NAME

Name: ————————— ID No.: ————————— Issued by: —————

Designation: ——————— Department: ——————— Date: ——————

3.6.3. Solids

    3.6.3.1. *Materials in kegs or drums.* The sampler sticks a sampled label to the selected keg/drum, then removes the lid and carefully, to avoid dust, undoes the plastic liner and then folds it back over the sides of the keg.

    The material should be examined for uniformity and visible contamination by turning the upper few inches over with a scoop. If the material appears to be non-uniform, the laboratory supervisor must be informed. Samples are then taken by withdrawing material with a scoop or sampling spear for "cored" samples. The caps of bottles containing hygroscopic material must be securely taped in position. Once the sample(s) has been taken, the sampler quickly folds the plastic fastener, and replaces the lid.

    3.6.3.2. *Materials in paper or plastic sacks or bags.* The sampler cleans a six-inch square area of the bag to remove dust/dirt; then using a sharp clean knife, cuts a small "V" in the centre of the clean area. A sampling scoop (open side uppermost) is pushed into the bag via the "V" leaving "U" shaped flap. The sample obtained is transferred to the pre-labelled sample bottle and examined for uniformity and visual contamination. He then repairs the tear by closing the flap and covering it with a piece of self-adhesive tape. QA label is affixed, signed and dated. For paper bags, immediately after the first sampling, transfer the material in a cleaned polybag followed by transfer on one pallet.

3.6.4. *Liquids.* The sampler ensures that the cap or closure is clean and free from dirt and water by wiping with a piece of rug/cloth. The closure is removed with the appropriate drum "key." A sample is then taken from about the middle of the container and transferred to an appropriate bottle.

    N.B. Viscous liquids, for example, Vitamin A requires mixing before the drum is opened.

    Note 3: Avoid banging or scraping the pipette against the inside of the drum to avoid the end breaks or splinters.

YOUR COMPANY NAME

Name: _____ ID No.: _____ Issued by: _____

Designation: _____ Department: _____ Date: _____

Materials, which are completely or partially frozen, must be melted entirely and mixed thoroughly before sampling. Drums to be thawed must have the closure loosened, then they should be moved into a suitable warm area.

When sampling is complete, the bulk container must be re-closed securely and any sample spillage around the opening should be wiped away.

If the bulk container headspace is normally purged with nitrogen, this must be re-flushed after sampling.

Drums of flammable liquids must not be brought into the store, that is, they must be sampled in the solvent store.

3.6.5. *Samples for microbiological analysis.* Explain that when taking samples intended for microbiological examination, extreme care must be exercised to avoid biological contamination of the sample, as this may invalidate the tests.

Although some of the details in Sections 3.3 through 3.6 still apply, it is important to observe the following additional points, peculiar to microbiological sampling.

Sterile sample bottle/lids and spatulas must be used; damaged or open bottles must not be used. These are provided by microbiological control laboratory.

For each container sampled, a fresh sterile spatula must be used to transfer sample from the container to the sterile bottle. The sampling should be performed under HEPA filters.

Ensure that hands and clothing do not come into contact with the product, the inside surfaces of the sample bottle, bottleneck, lid and sampling end of spatula. If a sterile spatula or bottle comes into contact with any other article, it must be discarded and fresh sterile item should be used.

If the material to be sampled is in unlined paper sack, wipe the surface when the incision is to be made with a little absolute alcohol, allow to dry, then cut a "V" shape with a sharp sterile blade, lift the flap and take the microbiological analysis sample with a sterile spatula, transferring into a labelled sterile bottle. When sufficient material has been taken, immediately seal the sample bottle with its sterile lid.

While sampling for microbiological analysis and chemical tests, always take the first sample for the microbiological

YOUR COMPANY NAME

Name: _____ ID No.: _____ Issued by: _____

Designation: _____ Department: _____ Date: _____

tests and seal that sample bottle immediately, once it has been filled. Then having taken the sample for chemical testing, the bulk container should be sealed as appropriate.

Sampling of water supplies is covered by a separate SOP and is the responsibility of microbiological control function.

All training carried out must be entered on the training log copy, which should be kept updated by both the trainee and the QA/QC manager.

QCT-03.3.1

Training of Conventional Procedures

YOUR COMPANY NAME

Name: _____ ID No.: _____ Issued by: _____

Designation: _____ Department: _____ Date: _____

Provide training to analyst responsible for the chemical testing.

PROCEDURE

The training of a chemist covers wide range of analytical techniques. The following chemical testing procedures have been covered in this training material:

1. Weighing
2. Volumetric techniques
3. Temperature measurement and control
4. Mechanical methods of separation
5. Limit tests
6. Determination of density and weight per millilitre
7. Physical observation
8. Testing to specification/practical work
9. Chromatographic techniques
    a. Thin-layer chromatography (TLC)
    b. High-performance liquid chromatography (HPLC)
    c. Gas chromatography
10. Spectroscopic techniques
    a. UV absorption and colorimetry
    b. Infrared methods
    c. Atomic absorption spectroscopy (AAS)
    d. Flame emission spectroscopy
11. Electrochemical techniques
    a. pH measurement and ion selective electrodes
    b. Potentiometric titrations

YOUR COMPANY NAME

Name: _____ ID No.: _____ Issued by: _____

Designation: _____ Department: _____ Date: _____

    c.   Biaperometric titrations (including Karl Fischer)
    d.   Automatic titrations
 12. Miscellaneous techniques
    a.   Polarimetry
    b.   Particle size analysis
    c.   Viscometry
    d.   Disintegration
    e.   Dissolution
    f.   Additional techniques

QCT-03.3.2

Training of Basic Analytical Techniques

YOUR COMPANY NAME

Name: _____ ID No.: _____ Issued by: _____

Designation: _____ Department: _____ Date: _____

WEIGHING

Explain the appropriate use of bench and analytical balances.

Mention the difference between bench-top and four-figure balances.

Emphasize that all balances must be used according to their SOPs especially in regard to the daily calibration and checking.

SOMETHING MORE ON THE USE OF THE ANALYTICAL BALANCE

1. Must be kept clean; otherwise samples may be contaminated and balance may be damaged.
2. Must balance or "tare" before weighing samples and, where further weighing is carried out, use the same balance each time.
3. Show the appropriate use of weighing bottles, and so on and the use of syringes, cylinders, and so on for weighing liquids. When electronic balances are used, the "tare" facility may be used to weigh materials directly into flasks, beakers, and so on.
4. Never overload balances.
5. Ensure that the fingers are dry when weighing glassware, or use tongs, and so on.
6. Close the doors gently.
7. Objects must be dried at the same temperature as the balance (air current and buoyancy effects).
8. Record all weightings directly into notebook in ink or take printouts wherever possible.
9. Consult senior analyst if any problems.

YOUR COMPANY NAME

Name: _____ ID No.: _____ Issued by: _____

Designation: _____ Department: _____ Date: _____

VOLUMETRIC TECHNIQUES

Explain when and how to use, including restrictions, the following:

1. Cylinder/pipette/burette/syringe
2. Volumetric flask/conical flask/beaker
3. Boiling tube/test tube/Nessler cylinder
4. Reflux/distillation
5. Concentrated/dilute solutions (especially with respect to SOPs)

Show how to use pipette fillers and/or bulbs; then allow the trainee to weigh several 10.0 mL aliquots pipetted out into a weighing bottle, and so on. Stress the importance of wiping outside of pipette with a dry tissue.

DEFINITIONS

Explain the important terms relating to volumetric analysis including the following:

1. End points and equivalence points
2. Indicators
3. pH
4. Upper and lower meniscus
5. mL
6. Equivalent
7. Factor
8. Molarity
9. % w/v, % w/w, ppm and their relationship
10. Assay, and so on
11. Non-aqueous titrations

USE OF BURETTE

Show how to use and read burette correctly for colourless and coloured liquids.
Show or explain effect of "greasy" burette on meniscus and its results. Also explain the use of burette cards or magnifier.
Explain the importance of using a clean burette and pipette.

YOUR COMPANY NAME

Name: _____ ID No.: _____ Issued by: _____

Designation: _____ Department: _____ Date: _____

TEMPERATURE MEASUREMENT AND CONTROL

Use of ordinary and standardized thermometers:
Explain the terms melting point and melting range.

1. The trainee should be shown how to determine melting point and melting range of a substance readily reduced to a powder using the apparatus in use in the laboratory, emphasizing on all the important points, that is, heating rate, height of sample column, addition of tube, and so on.
2. The trainee should carry out suitable melting range determinations.

HEATING

1. Explain use of water, steam and oil baths.
2. Explain use of burners and when to use hotplates, isomantles, and so on.
3. Explain use of ovens, vacuum ovens and muffle furnace. According to SOPs, hazards of flammable solvents in ovens should be emphasized, for example, TLC plates, and so on.

COOLING

1. Show from where to get ice and use of ice bowls, and so on.
2. Special use of "freezing mixture," for example, ice/salt and solid CO_2.
3. Use of desiccators for cooling apparatus.

MECHANICAL METHODS OF SEPARATION

1. Explain and show use of different types of filters including paper and Buchner, and sintered glass with vacuum, including transfer techniques.
2. The trainee should carry out quantitative transfer exercise.
3. Explain and show use of separating funnels, including cleaning procedures and potential hazards.
4. Trainee to carry out simple extraction exercise.
5. Explain and show the use of centrifuge and use it to separate a suspension. Cover the topic of the hazards of using flammable solvents during training of centrifuge.

YOUR COMPANY NAME

Name: _____ ID No.: _____ Issued by: _____

Designation: _____ Department: _____ Date: _____

LIMIT TESTS

Explain the uses of limit test and their limitations. Two types of limit test are mainly in use: BP/EP limit test and USP-type limit test. Where both types of limit tests are used, both should be carried out by the trainee, otherwise carry out just the older BP limit tests.

LIMIT TEST FOR CHLORIDE

Basis of the test will include Br, I, CN, CNS and any other acid radicals that give silver salts insoluble in nitric acid.

  a. Using appropriate methods of analysis, explain how to carry out limit test, especially calculations.
  b. The trainee should carry out chloride determinations on suitable samples or known solution including several standards to confirm reproducibility.

LIMIT TEST FOR SULPHATE

Basis of the test includes reason for seeding reagent rather than just barium chloride.

  a. Difference between opalescence and turbidity.
  b. Explain how to carry out limit test, especially calculations.
  c. The trainee should carry out sulphate determination on suitable samples or solution.

LIMIT TEST FOR IRON

Basis of tests: thioglycollic acid and thiocyanate (only used for substances that precipitate in alkali—very rarely).

  a. Using appropriate methods of analysis, explain how to carry out limit test, especially calculations.
  b. Trainee to carry out iron determination on suitable samples or solution.

YOUR COMPANY NAME

Name: _____ ID No.: _____ Issued by: _____

Designation: _____ Department: _____ Date: _____

Limit Tests for Lead or Heavy Metals

Basis of tests include reasons for acetic acid, cyanide, burn sugar and importance of buffer and correct quantities of reagents in the EP method. Explain the term "Heavy Metals."

    a. Using appropriate methods of analysis, explain how to carry out the limit tests, especially calculations.
    b. The trainee should carry out lead and heavy metal determinations on suitable samples or solution as discussed in QAS-022.

Limit Test for Sulphated Ash (or Ash)

    a. Explain sulphated ash test.
    b. Explain use and care of platinum dishes.
    c. Explain how to carry out the limit test, emphasizing the important points, that is, hazards, must add H_2SO_4 in fume cupboard, correct heating and importance of cooling times.
    d. Trainee to carry out determination on suitable samples.

Limit for Loss on Drying

    a. Explain the reason for test and methods for carrying it out. Emphasize the preparation of the sample and the importance of adequate cooling times.
    b. Ensure that the trainee understands what is "dried to constant weight."
    c. Trainee to carry out at least duplicate determinations on suitable samples (one of which at least should be hygroscopic when dry).

DETERMINATION OF WEIGHT PER MILLILITRE DENSITY/SOLIDS

    a. Explain use of density bottle or pycnometer and the care required to handle them.
    b. Emphasize the importance of temperature on the result.
    c. Trainee to carry out weight per millilitre on a suitable liquid.
    d. Trainee to carry out a determination, if required.

YOUR COMPANY NAME

Name: _____ ID No.: _____ Issued by: _____

Designation: _____ Department: _____ Date: _____

PHYSICAL OBSERVATIONS

   a. Emphasize the possible hazards involved with toxic materials and what
      precautions may be needed to be taken.
   b. Explain the importance of these tests with regard to approval of material
      for sale or use and assessment of any deterioration on storage.
   c. Include methods used for the determination of colour and clarity of sol-
      ids and liquids, for example, colour charts, alpha units, and so on.

QCT-03.3.3

Training of Chromatographic Techniques

YOUR COMPANY NAME

Name: _____ ID No.: _____ Issued by: _____

Designation: _____ Department: _____ Date: _____

TESTING TO SPECIFICATION/PRACTICAL WORK

1. Provide the trainee with some practical work of similar nature to that which he/she will be carrying out (preferably something that has already been examined so that the trainee's accuracy can be assessed) or get the trainee to test several samples of increasing complexity ensuring that relevant methods of analysis have been dealt with.
2. Emphasize the importance of the following methods/procedures and also of time management/planning when carrying out tests.
3. Stress precautions are necessary when dealing with hygroscopic and very toxic materials. Explain what to do in the event of test failure and the procurement of further samples if necessary. Explain the use of reference and "check" samples.

CHROMATOGRAPHIC TECHNIQUES

1. Explain that separation of the variation is achieved in the rate at which different components of a mixture migrate through a stationary phase under the influence of a mobile phase and how a chromatogram is obtained.
2. Explain how a sample may be tentatively identified by virtue of its Rf value in TLC or its retention time GC and HPLC, whatever the instrument available.
3. Show for GC and HPLC how the efficiency of a column can be calculated and how inefficient column can affect a separation giving false results. Calculate the Plate No. and asymmetry factors for some pre-run chromatograms.
4. Explain differences between TLC, GC and HPLC and the types of compounds, which can be examined by each method.

YOUR COMPANY NAME

Name: _____ ID No.: _____ Issued by: _____

Designation: _____ Department: _____ Date: _____

THIN-LAYER CHROMATOGRAPHY

a. Explain the basic principles and procedures used, including hazards and any special precautions necessary, for example, for photo/air-sensitive compounds.
b. Explain limitations, for example, semi-quantitative technique, limit of detection, spot size, and so on, preparation of sample and standard solutions and relationship of percentage of impurity to μg spotted.
c. Explain or show different methods of visualization and methods of assessment of spots.
d. Cover during the explanation, use and care of μL (microlitre) syringe.
e. Trainee to carry out simple TLC method.

HIGH-PERFORMANCE LIQUID CHROMATOGRAPHY

A liquid chromatograph consists of the following parts:

a. Reservoir containing the mobile phase
b. Pump to force the mobile phase through the system at high pressure
c. Injector to introduce the sample into the mobile phase
d. Chromatographic column
e. Detector
f. Data collection device such as computer, integrator or recorder

Using the relevant SOP, manufacturer's manual and the instruments, explain the action and uses of the solvent, pumps, column, detector and any integrating/computing device used.

Include in the explanation: the types of solvents used for different separation, purity of solvents and importance of de-gassing; the connection care and use of columns; cleaning and storage procedures, and so on, use of sample valves, auto sampler, and so on; use of detector and pump and the potential hazards involved (flammability of solvents, high pressure, and so on UV radiation); use of pumps for isocratic or solvent; flow programming. For a schematic presentation of an HPLC system see Figure 3.1.

HPLC PUMPING SYSTEM

1. HPLC pumping system delivers metered amounts of mobile phase from the solvent reservoirs to the column through high-pressure tubing and fittings.

YOUR COMPANY NAME

Name: _____ ID No.: _____ Issued by: _____

Designation: _____ Department: _____ Date: _____

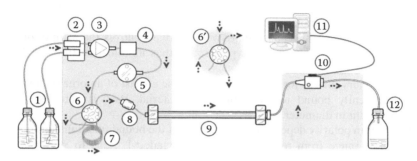

FIGURE 3.1 Schematic representation of an HPLC unit. (1) Solvent reservoirs, (2) solvent degasser, (3) gradient valve, (4) mixing vessel for delivery of the mobile phase, (5) high-pressure pump, (6) switching valve in inject position, (6′) switching valve in load position, (7) sample injection loop, (8) pre-column (guard column), (9) analytical column, (10) detector (i.e., IR, UV), (11) data acquisition, (12) waste or fraction collector.

    2. Pumps can be programmed to vary the ratio of mobile phase components, as is required for gradient chromatography or can use only one mobile phase as required for isocratic.

    3. Operating pressure up to 5000 PSI or higher with flow rates up to 10 mL/min is typical. Pumps used for quantitative analysis should be constructed of materials inert to corrosive mobile phase at a constant rate with minimal fluctuation over extended periods of time.

INJECTORS

Compounds to be chromatographed are injected into the mobile phase, either manually by syringe or loop injectors, or automatically by auto samplers.

COLUMNS

    1. For most pharmaceutical analyses, separation is achieved by partition of compounds in the test solution between the mobile and stationary phases.

    2. Systems consisting of polar stationary phases and non-polar mobile phases are described as normal phase, while the other type, polar mobile phases and non-polar stationary phases are called reverse-phase chromatography.

YOUR COMPANY NAME

Name: _____ ID No.: _____ Issued by: _____

Designation: _____ Department: _____ Date: _____

3. Partition chromatography is almost always used for hydrocarbon-soluble compounds of molecular weight less than 1000.
4. Making the mobile phase more or less polar controls the affinity of a compound for the stationary phase, and thus its retention time on the column.
5. Stationary phases for modern reverse-phase consist of an organic phase chemically bound to silica or other material. Particles are usually 3–10 μm in diameter.
6. Column polarity depends on the polarity of the bound functional groups, which range from relatively non-polar octadecyl silane to very polar nitrile groups.
7. Column may be heated to give more efficient separation.
8. IEC is used to separate water-soluble, ionizable compounds of molecular weight less than 1500. The stationary phases are usually synthetic organic resin.
9. Cation-exchange resin contains negatively charged active sites and is used to separate basic substances such as amines.
10. Anion-exchange resins have positively charged active sites for separation of compounds with negatively charged groups such as phosphate, sulphonate or carboxylate groups.

DETECTORS

1. Spectrophotometric detectors:
   a. This type of detectors consists of a flow-cell mounted at the end of the column.
   b. A beam of UV radiation passes through the flow cell and into the detector. As compounds elute from the column, they pass through the cell and absorb the radiation, resulting in measurable energy level changes. Fixed, variable and multi-wavelength detectors are widely available.
2. Differential refractometer detector:
   a. Such a detector measures the difference between the refractive index of the mobile phase alone and that of the mobile phase containing the chromatographed compounds as it emerges from the column.
   b. Refractive index detectors are used to detect non-UV absorbing compounds.
3. Fluorometric detectors:

YOUR COMPANY NAME

Name: _____ ID No.: _____ Issued by: _____

Designation: _____ Department: _____ Date: _____

    a.   This type of detector is sensitive to compounds that are inherently fluorescent or that can be converted to fluorescent derivatives either by chemical transformation of the compound or by coupling with fluorescent reagents at specific functional groups.

4. Potentiometric or polarographic electrochemical detectors:

    a.   These detectors are useful for the quantization of species that can be oxidized or reduced at a working electrode.

    b.   These detectors require conducting mobile phases free of dissolved oxygen and reducible metal ions.

    c.   A pulseless pump must be used, and care must be taken to ensure that the pH, ionic strength and temperature of the mobile phase remain constant.

5. Electrochemical detectors with carbon-paste electrodes:

    a.   Such a detector may be used to measure nanogram quantities of easily oxidized compounds, notably phenols and catechols.

6. Mobile phase polarity can be varied by addition of some components.

7. Trainee to carry out simple HPLC separation.

SOLVENTS AND REAGENTS

1. The mobile phase composition significantly influences chromatographic performance and the resolution of compounds in the mixture being chromatographed.

2. For accurate quantitative work, high purity reagents and HPLC grade, organic solvents must be used.

3. Water of suitable quality should have low conductivity and low UV absorption, appropriate to the intended use.

DATA HANDLING AND INTERPRETATION

    a. Show how a chromatogram can be obtained on a recorder and how to measure the area or height of peak manually (e.g., ht × w 1/2, etc.).

    b. Explain how an integrator/computer detects and measures peaks.

    c. Using the manufacturer manual, explain how to generate methods that will calculate the area or height of peaks and present the results in a suitable format.

    d. Emphasize the effect that the various parameters can have on the results, for example, peak thresholds, baseline and area sensitivities, attenuation,

YOUR COMPANY NAME

Name: _____ ID No.: _____ Issued by: _____

Designation: _____ Department: _____ Date: _____

     and so on and that the values set for various analyses must not be changed without permission.

  e. Ensure that the trainee understands the difference between qualitative and quantitative work.

  f. Introduce the use of external and internal standard "assay" methods and how to set up and use them.

  g. Explain the importance of using the same conditions for sample and standard and similarity of areas.

  h. Ensure that the trainee understands the importance of obtaining reproducible peak areas/heights before commencing analysis.

  i. Emphasize that there are many problems that can occur with a determination, for example, drifting base lines or retention times, noisy detection, and so on.

  j. Always refer to standard or reference chromatograms or previous analyses to ensure that what is obtained is correct.

  k. Always ask if in doubt, for example, loss of efficiency, peak splitting, source of noise, and so on.

  l. Trainee to carry out a simple chromatographic separation.

GAS CHROMATOGRAPHY

A gas chromatography consists of a carrier gas source, an injection port, column, detector and recording device. The injection port, column and detector are temperature controlled. The typical carrier gas is helium, nitrogen or hydrogen, depending on the column and detector in use.

SAMPLE INJECTION

Compounds to be chromatographed, either in solution or as gases, are injected into the carrier gas stream at the injection port to enter the column. Compounds are separated according to the difference in their capacity factor, which in turn depends upon vapour pressure and degree of interaction with the stationary phase.

TYPES OF COLUMNS

  a. Packed columns: Packed columns are made of glass or metal and are 1–3 m in length with internal diameter ranging from 2 to 4 mm. The liquid stationary phase is deposited on a finely divided inert solid support

YOUR COMPANY NAME

Name: _____ ID No.: _____ Issued by: _____

Designation: _____ Department: _____ Date: _____

such as diatomaceous earth, porous polymer that is packed into a column that is typically 2–4 mm in internal diameter.

b. Capillary columns: Capillary columns are usually made of fused silica, and are typically 0.2–0.53 mm in internal diameter and 5–60 m in length. The liquid stationary phase, which is sometimes chemically bonded to the inner surface, is 0.1–1.0 μm thick. Although the non-polar stationary phase may be up to 5 μm thick.

INJECTORS

Sample injection devices range from simple syringes to fully programmable automatic injectors. The amount of sample that can be injected into capillary column is small compared to the amount that can be injected into the packed columns.

Headspace injectors are equipped with a thermostatically controlled sample-heating chamber. Solid or liquid samples in tightly closed containers are heated in the chamber for a fixed period of time. The injector automatically introduces a fixed amount of the headspace in the sample container into the gas chromatography.

DETECTORS

Flame ionization detectors are used for most pharmaceutical analysis. These detectors have a wide linear range and are sensitive to most organic compounds.

Other types of detectors used are

a. Thermal conductivity detector
b. Electron capture detector
c. Nitrogen–phosphorus
d. Mass spectrometric detectors

PROCEDURE

Using the relevant SOP or manufacturer's manual and the instrument itself, explain the action and use of

a. Mobile phase (carries gas) pressure and flow control system and their effect on the chromatogram.
b. Sample injection system—normally hot zone injection, include column injection and split or split less injection systems for capillary columns if necessary.

YOUR COMPANY NAME

Name: _____ ID No.: _____ Issued by: _____

Designation: _____ Department: _____ Date: _____

   c. Column includes preparation and packing of columns; types of support
and stationary phase and their selection; fitting and removal of columns
in instrument; use of capillary columns (if available); importance of correct oven temperature and its effect on the chromatogram; the use of
isothermal or temperature programmed runs.

   d. Detector—short sessions on the various detectors in use in the laboratory which could include

     1. Thermal conductivity detector—For example, minimum detectable
quantity 10^{-9} gs^{-1}; linear range 10^4; temperature limit 450°C;
temperature

     2. Flow sensitive: Non-destructive, useful for water and certain gases
(CO_2, O_2 etc.); for example, always need gases flowing before on.

     3. Flame Ionization Detector—Minimum detectable quantity 10^{-11}
gs^{-1}; linear range 10^7; temperature limit 400°C; destructive excellent stability; most common detector for the vast majority of compounds; hazards of air/hydrogen mixtures; poor response to water,
formic acid and inorganic gases; modifications to give nitrogen
phosphorous detectors using alkali halide beads sensitivity to P & N
10^{-12} gs^{-1}.

   e. Recording device—Use of amplification/attenuation to get peaks on
scale; recorder ranges.

   f. Sample introduction—Use of microlitre syringes and gas sampling
valves or syringes.

   g. Trainee to carry out a simple chromatographic separation.

   h. Columns must be conditioned before use until the baseline is stable. This
may be done by operation at temperature below the maximum of the
column temperature for about 4 hours.

   i. Assays require quantitative comparison of one chromatogram with another.
A major source of error is irreproducibility in the amount of sample injected,
notably when manual injections are made with a syringe. The effect of
variability can be minimized by addition of internal standard solutions.
See the schematic diagram of a typical gas chromatograph in Figure 3.2.

   j. Automatic injectors greatly improve the reproducibility of sample injections and reduce the need for internal standards.

DATA HANDLING AND INTERPRETATION

   a. Show how a chromatogram can be obtained on a recorder and how to
measure the area or height of the peak manually (e.g., ht × w (1/2), etc.).

YOUR COMPANY NAME

Name: _____ ID No.: _____ Issued by: _____

Designation: _____ Department: _____ Date: _____

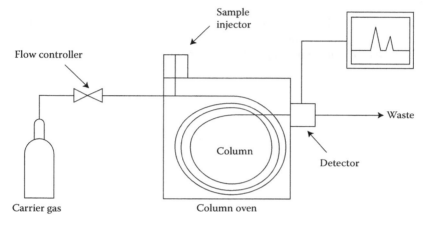

FIGURE 3.2 Schematic diagram of a gas chromatograph.

- b. Explain how an integrator/computer detects and measures peaks.
- c. Using the manufacturer's manual, explain how to generate methods that will calculate the areas or height of peaks and present the results in a suitable format. Emphasize the effect that various data handling parameters can have on the results, for example, peak width, thresholds, baseline setting/peak skinning and that the values set for various analyses should not be changed without permission.
- d. Ensure that the trainee understands the difference between qualitative and quantitative work (use of retention time, etc.).
- e. Introduce use of external and internal standard "assay" methods and how to set up and use them. Emphasize the importance of using the same conditions for sample and standard to obtain similar areas.
- f. Ensure that the trainee understands the importance of obtaining reproducible peak heights/areas before commencing analysis.
- g. Emphasize that there are many problems that can occur with a determination giving poor results, for example, drifting baselines and retention times, leaky columns and septa, noisy detectors, and so on. It is important for the trainee to recognize and deal with simple faults. Always refer to standard or reference chromatograms, if available, to ensure what is obtained appears correct.
- h. Cover the use of autosamplers if available.

YOUR COMPANY NAME

Name: _____ ID No.: _____ Issued by: _____

Designation: _____ Department: _____ Date: _____

SAMPLE PREPARATION

   a. Ensure that the trainee understands that a sample must be volatile and
      thermally stable below 400°C.
   b. Trainee to carry out simple chromatographic separation.

QCT-03.3.4
Spectroscopic Techniques

YOUR COMPANY NAME

Name: _____ ID No.: _____ Issued by: _____

Designation: _____ Department: _____ Date: _____

UV ABSORPTION AND COLORIMETRY

1. Explain absorbencies and its relationship to percentage transmission and transmittance.
2. Explain briefly the Beer–Lambert law and its main limitations producing curved calibration graphs, for example,
   a. Can only be used for dilute solutions.
   b. Chemical interaction may interfere.
   c. Importance of measuring absorbance at the maximum and effects of slit width and astray light for sharp peaks, and so on.

BEER–LAMBERT LAW

The law states that the quantity of light absorbed by a substance dissolved in a non-absorbent solvent is directly proportional to the concentration of the substance and the path length of the light through the solution.

Beer's law is commonly written in the form $A = \varepsilon c l$, where A is the absorbance, c is the concentration in moles per litre, l is the path length in centimeters, and ε is a constant of proportionality known as the molar extinction coefficient.

3. Explain the use of UV/visible spectrophotometer using relevant SOPs.
   a. Emphasize the differences between glass and quartz cells and the importance of their handling and cleaning.
   b. Importance of using the same solvent throughout determination.
   c. What to do in the event of spillages in instrument, and so on.
4. Explain special precautions to be taken with photosensitive materials, for example, use of amber glassware.
5. Emphasize the importance of temperature on non-aqueous solvents.
6. Show how to prepare a simple calibration curve.

YOUR COMPANY NAME

Name: _____ ID No.: _____ Issued by: _____

Designation: _____ Department: _____ Date: _____

7. Trainee to carry out a suitable colorimetric exercise.
8. Trainee to carry out a UV determination on a suitable substance and/or calculate specific absorbance of reference substance.

INFRARED SPECTROPHOTOMETRY

1. Explain how molecules can absorb infrared radiation causing changes in their vibrational energy.
2. This absorption can be measured and is related to the various groups within the molecule each of which will absorb at characteristic frequencies.
3. Based on the above, show the positions on an IR spectrum where various functional groups (e.g., –OH, –CH3, –C=O, –CH$_2$, etc.) occur and how IR can be used as a "fingerprint" for identification and for structure evaluation.
4. Mention its use for quantitative purposes.
5. Explain the use of IR spectrophotometer using relevant SOP.
6. Explain and show various methods of sample preparation.
7. Explain and show the effects on the spectrum of an improperly prepared disc (powdery), the effect of water and the effect of too little and too much sample present.
8. Show how to compare the spectrum with a reference spectrum and what to do in the event of a discrepancy.
9. Trainee to carry out two IR identity tests using thin-film and KBr disc technique on suitable samples. A typical apparatus of IR spectrophotometer is shown in Figure 3.3.

ATOMIC ABSORPTION SPECTROMETRY

Principles

1. Atomic absorption spectrometry (AAS) is based on absorption of electromagnetic radiation in the visible and UV regions of the spectrum by atoms, resulting in changes in electronic structure.
2. This absorption is proportional to the concentration of the atoms in a manner closely resembling the Beer–Lambert law for molecular absorption (see UV/visible spectrophotometry).
3. The absorption can be measured by passing radiation characteristic of a particular element through an atomic vapour of the sample. This atomic vapour is produced by vaporizing the sample either by aspiration of a solution into a flame or by evaporation from an electrically heated

YOUR COMPANY NAME

Name: _____ ID No.: _____ Issued by: _____

Designation: _____ Department: _____ Date: _____

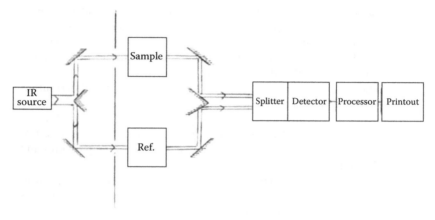

FIGURE 3.3 Schematic diagram to show a typical apparatus of infrared spectrophotometer.

surface. Figure 3.4 shows the principle of function of atomic absorption spectrophotometer.

INSTRUMENTATION

1. Using the relevant instrument SOP, explain the trainee, the operation of the spectrometer for determining the metallic impurities in a sample.

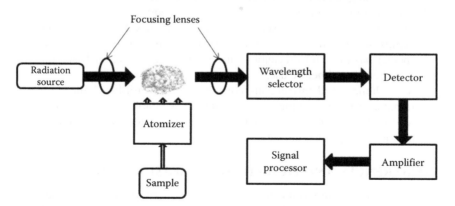

FIGURE 3.4 Schematic diagram to show the function of atomic absorption spectrophotometer.

YOUR COMPANY NAME

Name: _____ ID No.: _____ Issued by: _____

Designation: _____ Department: _____ Date: _____

2. Ensure that the trainee is shown and explained how to set up and use:
   a. The sharp-line radiation source characteristic of the element of inter-est, that is, usually a hollow cathode lamp (two types available).
   b. Single and multi-element: although an electrodeless discharge source is used this should be covered.
   c. The means of introducing the sample—that is, the nebulizer/burner system and its adjustment.
   d. Cover the use and operation of the gas system and the hazards asso-ciated with that of acetylene and nitrous oxide flames, that is, UV emission and the importance of cylinder and working pressures and flow rates.
   e. If the instrument has calibration facility, its use, together with appropriate calibration solutions which allow direct display of ele-ment concentration, should be covered.
   f. It is very important to cover emergency shutdown procedures, that is, what to do in the event of a gas system failure and the importance of preventing gas from escaping via the nebulizer drain tube and receiver.

SAMPLE PREPARATION AND VAPORIZATION

1. As most AA measurement are concerned with determination of very small quantities of metals (usually ppm), it is very important that all apparatus is thoroughly cleaned before use (i.e., by washing with acid, etc., and thor-ough rinsing) and that all reagents used, be of suitable purity.
2. Although most samples may be aspirated as aqueous solutions, some-times (to achieve better sensitivity or remove interfering substances) metals are determined as suitable complexes in organic solvents. The special hazards and precautions necessary when using such solutions must be covered before use.
3. Most flame-based instruments consume several millilitre samples per minute; sufficient sample must therefore be available to enable a steady reading to be taken (an advantage of flameless systems is that consider-ably less sample is required).

INTERFERENCES AND QUANTITATIVE MEASUREMENTS

1. It is also very important that any calibration solution used must match the sample solution as closely as possible to avoid any errors caused by matrix effects.

YOUR COMPANY NAME

Name: _____ ID No.: _____ Issued by: _____

Designation: _____ Department: _____ Date: _____

2. Interference in absorption measurement can arise from both chemical and physical sources.
3. Chemical effects include stable compound formation and ionization, both of which decrease the population of free atoms in the sample giving low absorbance.
4. Compound formation usually occurs between alkaline earth metals and anions, such as silicate and phosphate.
5. Interference can usually be prevented by addition of strontium or lanthanum salts as "releasing" agents.
6. Adding an easily ionizable metal, for example, lithium or sodium that acts as a "buffer," can sometimes prevent ionization.
7. Physical interference may arise from using too strong solutions when solids may block the burner or by changes in aspiration rate due to viscosity or surface tension of solutions changing.
8. Quantitative measurements may be made by using a freshly prepared calibration curve, which has been zeroed against a blank solution, or by using the method of standard addition. In both cases, operating conditions must first be optimized to obtain the maximum possible response. Concentration of samples should be selected, where possible, to take into account the linear working range of the element being determined (most instrument manuals give guidelines on operating conditions and working concentrations for metals and these should be consulted where appropriate).

TRAINEE ASSESSMENT

The trainee should carry out a suitable atomic absorption determination used in the laboratory, preferably on a previously analysed sample as discussed in the corresponding SOP.

FLAME EMISSION SPECTROMETRY

1. Principles: Electromagnetic radiation in the visible and UV regions is emitted by some atoms when they are "excited" in a flame.
2. Some elements emit light more readily than others, notably the alkali metals; and this technique is often used in preference to AA, for metals.
3. The basic instrumentation is very similar to that used for AA without the hallow cathode lamp (most AA instruments can, in fact, operate as emission spectrometers).

YOUR COMPANY NAME

Name: _____ ID No.: _____ Issued by: _____

Designation: _____ Department: _____ Date: _____

4. The trainee must be shown how to operate correctly whichever type of instrument is in use in the laboratory.
5. Demonstration should be done using the relevant instrument SOP, emphasizing the hazards associated with instruments using gas flames.
6. If compressed gases are used, the trainee must be first made familiar with hazards and safety procedures.
7. As with AA, the trainee must be fully conversant with emergency shutdown procedures.

SAMPLE PREPARATION AND VAPORIZATION

1. As most AA measurement are concerned with determination of very small quantities of metals (usually ppm), it is very important that all apparatus is thoroughly cleaned before use (i.e., by washing with acid, etc., and thorough rinsing) and that all reagents used, be of suitable purity.
2. Although most samples may be aspirated as aqueous solutions, sometimes (to achieve better sensitivity or remove interfering substances) metals are determined as suitable complexes in organic solvents. The special hazards and precautions necessary when using such solutions must be covered before use.
3. Most flame-based instruments consume several millilitre samples per minute; sufficient sample must therefore be available to enable a steady reading to be taken (an advantage of flameless systems is that considerably less sample is required).

INTERFERENCE AND QUANTITATIVE MEASUREMENTS

1. It is also very important that any calibration solution used must match the sample solution as closely as possible to avoid any errors caused by matrix effects.
2. Interference in absorption measurement can arise from both chemical and physical sources.
3. Chemical effects include stable compound formation and ionization, both of which decrease the population of free atoms in the sample giving low absorbance.
4. Compound formation usually occurs between alkaline earth metals and anions, such as silicate and phosphate.

YOUR COMPANY NAME

Name: _____ ID No.: _____ Issued by: _____

Designation: _____ Department: _____ Date: _____

5. Interference can usually be prevented by addition of strontium or lanthanum salts as "releasing" agents.
6. Adding an easily ionizable metal, for example, lithium or sodium that acts as a "buffer," can sometimes prevent ionization.
7. Physical interference may arise from using too strong solutions when solids may block the burner or by changes in aspiration rate due to viscosity or surface tension of solutions changing.
8. Quantitative measurements may be made by using a freshly prepared calibration curve, which has been zeroed against a blank solution, or by using the method of standard addition. In both cases, operating conditions must first be optimized to obtain the maximum possible response.
9. Concentration of samples should be selected, where possible, to take into account the linear working range of the element being determined (most instrument manuals give guidelines on operating conditions and working concentrations for metals and these should be consulted where appropriate).

TRAINEE ASSESSMENT

The trainee should carry out a suitable flame photometric determination use in the laboratory, preferably on a previously analysed sample as discussed in corresponding SOP.

QCT-03.3.5

Electrochemical Techniques

YOUR COMPANY NAME

Name: _____ ID No.: _____ Issued by: _____

Designation: _____ Department: _____ Date: _____

pH MEASUREMENT AND ION-SELECTIVE ELECTRODES

1. Explain how the potential of a galvanic cell usually measured at zero current, is governed by the potential of an indicator electrode which responds to change in the concentration (activity) of the species being measured.
2. The potential of the electrodes is being measured against that of a reference electrode whose potential is independent of the solution or concentration.
3. As a guide, explain what pH is and how it is a measure of the acidity or alkalinity of an aqueous solution.
4. Using the appropriate SOP, show how a pH meter can be used to measure the pH or mV potential of a solution.
5. Emphasize the care and use of reference and indicator electrodes and explain how to check that they are satisfactory before use.
6. Address the necessity for standardizing pH meters with buffer solutions (whose pH does not vary much with concentration), the importance of temperature control of the solutions being measured and how it can affect the pH and the need to have a homogenous sample and allowing the reading to stabilize.
7. Explain that certain indicator electrodes are highly selective in their response, that is, the potential obtained is a function of the concentration of one type of ion only or of a small number of types. Such electrodes are frequently known as ion-selective electrodes.
8. The trainee should calibrate the pH metre and prepare a suitable solution and measure its pH.
9. If required, the trainee should carry out a suitable determination using an ion-selective electrode method. In this case, the trainee must also be shown the necessity for reducing interferences.

YOUR COMPANY NAME

Name: _____ ID No.: _____ Issued by: _____

Designation: _____ Department: _____ Date: _____

POTENTIOMETER TITRATIONS, IF AVAILABLE

1. Explain to the trainee that when a sample is highly coloured or "dirty" or when the end point is indistinct, it is virtually impossible to use an indicator to determine the end point of a titration.
2. In this case it is often possible to determine the end point by monitoring the change in potential of an indicator electrode against that of a reference electrode, which responds to one of the reactants or products (in mV) or the pH recorded against volume of titrant added gives a characteristic "S-shaped" curve. The mid-point of the inflection of this curve is the end-point of the titration.
3. Explain to the trainee that the end point can be determined in several ways:
   a. By graphical means
   b. From the plotted curve
   c. By mathematical means
   d. Or using the "second-differential" method
4. Show the trainee how to connect indicator and reference electrodes to the pH metre or mV metre to be used and how to assemble the titration vessel, burette, electrodes, and so on, so that a titration can be carried out.
5. The trainee should carry out a suitable titration, determining the end-point by potentiometric means.

BIAMPEROMETRIC TITRATIONS

1. Explain to the trainee that these types of titrations are similar to polarographic or amperometric titrations but these use two identical stationary electrodes (usually platinum) across which a constant potential of between 10 and 500 mV is applied.
2. The equivalence point is marked by a sudden rise in current from zero (normally encountered and sometimes called "dead-stop" end-point) or by either a decrease to zero or a minimum at or near zero current.
3. The platinum electrodes assume the roles of anode and cathode and, in all cases, current flows in the cell only if there is a significant concentration of both the oxidized and reduced forms of one of the reactants.

KARL FISCHER TITRATIONS

1. This is perhaps one of the most common methods using biamperometric end point. Explain the hazards and limitations of the method, especially

YOUR COMPANY NAME

Name: _____ ID No.: _____ Issued by: _____

Designation: _____ Department: _____ Date: _____

the importance of protection from water, and the precautions necessary when titrating ketones, bases, acids, and so on.

2. Explain how the Karl Fischer (KF) reagent can be used to titrate small amounts of water either directly to a "dead-stop" end point or via back titration when an excess of KF reagent is titrated with a standard water solution and how to calculate the percentage water content from the volumes of KF reagent/standard water obtained in the determination.

3. Using the relevant instrument SOP, show how to carry out a water determination and, if required, how to standardize the reagents used.

4. The trainee should carry out a water determination on a suitable substance.

AUTOMATIC TITRATIONS

1. Explain to the trainee that titrations can also be automated and many laboratories have some form of apparatus for carrying out automatic titrations, that is, that generally the addition of titrate and ion of the end point is carried out by the instrument.

2. Some automatic titrators can also calculate assay results with the help of information supplied by the operator and can also present titration curves (volume versus mV or pH) if required.

3. If available within the laboratory, the trainees must be shown how to operate the automatic titrators using the relevant instrument SOP. Other important points like changing and standardizing titrants, safety aspects must also be addressed, for example, if flammable or toxic solutions are used, connection of electrodes must be checked, and so on.

4. If required, the trainee should carry out one or more titrations of suitable materials.

QCT-03.3.6

Dissolution Test

YOUR COMPANY NAME

Name: _____ ID No.: _____ Issued by: _____

Designation: _____ Department: _____ Date: _____

In the pharmaceutical industry, dissolution is defined as the amount of drug substance that goes into solution per unit time under standardized conditions of liquid/solid interface, temperature and solvent composition.

Dissolution is considered one of the most important QC tests performed on pharmaceutical dosage forms. It is a compendial method used to measure a drug's rate of release from its dosage form. As a matter of fact, it is a complement to other analytical assays (potency and related substances) that characterize the dosage form.

The factors triggering need of dissolution test are as follows:

a. For lot release and to measure lot-to-lot variability in routine QC analysis
b. Optimization of drug delivery rate during development studies
c. To estimate release and absorption rates in humans after an *in vitro–in vivo* correlation is established
d. To study the effects of time/temperature/humidity on the dosage form during stability studies of the product
e. To compare one dosage form to another (different formulations, different processes, analysis of competitor's samples)

1. Explain the term "Dissolution" with reference to active ingredient, controlled/sustained release and dissolution profile.
2. Type of dissolution apparatus: The dissolution test method involves immersing the dosage unit in a suitable medium, which is kept in motion at a constant speed; the drug substance is extracted from the dosage unit and dissolves in the medium. Explain to the trainee that dissolution of a tablet may be carried out in several ways:
   a. By using the BP apparatus 1/USP type-1 method of round-bottomed vessels with rotating baskets

YOUR COMPANY NAME

Name: _____ ID No.: _____ Issued by: _____

Designation: _____ Department: _____ Date: _____

    b.   By using the BP apparatus 2/USP type-2 method of round-bottomed vessels with rotating paddles

3. Apparatus 2 is generally preferred for immediate release due to ease of use, reproducibility, hydrodynamics and general acceptance.

4. By using the relevant SOP explain how the different types of dissolution systems work and are operated.

5. Dissolution is measured below saturation, at 37°C in water- or aqueous-based buffers (pH range of 1–7) in a dissolution apparatus under precisely controlled mechanical and operational parameters.

6. Attention should be drawn to the need to de-aerate all dissolution media before use, the importance of volume dissolution, temperature of the media (evaporation effects) and of rotation speed of paddles/baskets.

7. Depending on the nature of the drug, the dissolution tests are conducted for various durations from 15 min to 24 h with appropriate sampling

8. Emphasize the importance of sampling technique in relation to sample probes; filtration and time (stagger sampling technique, if necessary, when using more than one dissolution bath).

9. The results of the dissolution analysis are reported as cumulated percent drug dissolved at specified time intervals.

10. The trainee should carry out a suitable dissolution exercise.

QCT-03.3.7
Miscellaneous Techniques

YOUR COMPANY NAME

Name: _____ ID No.: _____ Issued by: _____

Designation: _____ Department: _____ Date: _____

POLARIMETRY

The measurement and interpretation of the polarization of transverse waves or electromagnetic waves is called polarimetry. Polarimetry is done on electromagnetic waves that have travelled through or have been reflected, refracted, or diffracted by some material in order to characterize that object.

Polarimeters serve to determine the concentration of samples with high accuracies where precision is critical.

A polarimeter consists of a polarized light source, an analyser, a graduated circle to measure the rotation angle, and sample tubes. The polarized light passes through the sample tube and exhibits angular rotation to the left (–) or right (+). On the opposite side, the polarizer is the analyser. Using optics, visual fields are manually adjusted by the user to measure the optical rotation angle.

1. Explain the terms optical and specific optical rotation including how they may be determined using a polarimeter.
2. Using the relevant SOP, explain how the particular polarimeter works and is operated.
3. Attention should be drawn to take care of the sample tubes, need for the solution to be clear and free from air bubbles, and the need for the tube end glasses to be clean.
4. Emphasize the importance of carrying out measurements at the specified temperature and of zeroing the instruments or recording the "blank" value before taking a measurement.
5. The trainee should prepare a solution of an appropriate sample in use in the laboratory (preferably a previously analysed sample), measure its optical rotation and determine its specific optical rotation.

YOUR COMPANY NAME

Name: _____ ID No.: _____ Issued by: _____

Designation: _____ Department: _____ Date: _____

PARTICLE SIZE ANALYSIS

1. The particle size or distribution of a product may be carried out in a number of ways—for example:
   a. Dry sieving, with and without brushing
   b. Wet sieving
   c. Machine sieving
2. Explain how results should be reported when using several sieves.
3. Explain how sieving analysis is carried out distinguishing between wet sieving, dry sieving with and without brushing and, if applicable, machine sieving and specially how results should be reported when using several sieves.
4. Emphasize the hazards that may be involved, for example, sieving a toxic or unpleasant substance or carrying out a wet mesh using a flammable organic solvent. It should be emphasized that these should be carried out in a fume cupboard.
5. The trainee should carry out suitable sieving exercise as discussed in the corresponding SOP.

SUPPOSITORY PENETRATION TESTER

Explain to the trainee the following points before using the instrument:

a. Thermostat setting must be at 37°C.
b. Water level in the water tank must be enough to cover the thermostat.
c. Ensure that the penetration rod is freely moving.
   1. Actuate the main switch of the heater-cum-water circulator.
   2. Heat the water up to 37°C ± 0.5°C.
   3. Close the three washed and cleaned testing tubes with the stoppers and fill each tube with about 5 mL of water at 37°C so that the level reaches the top edge of the constriction.
   4. Place one of the suppositories to be tested in each of the three testing tubes and adjust the resting position on the constriction without pressure with the help of inner guide tubes.
   5. The rubber stoppers at the top opening of the testing tubes hold the inner guide tubes at the desired height.
   6. Insert and lower in each of the inner guide tube a penetration rod until its point rests on the test sample.

YOUR COMPANY NAME

Name: _____ ID No.: _____ Issued by: _____

Designation: _____ Department: _____ Date: _____

7. When the penetration rod has pierced the sample and the point of the penetration rod is visible in the constriction of the test tube, the test is completed.

VISCOMETRY

1. Explain to the trainee that the viscosity of a liquid or solution may be carried out by two main ways.
   a. By measuring the time that a measured volume of liquid takes to flow through a capillary tube under standard conditions (U-tube or suspended-level type viscometer)
   b. By measuring the torque produced when a cylinder or disk is rotated through a liquid (Brook field)
2. Explain the units of viscosity and the difference between kinematics and dynamic viscosity and the importance of temperature control.
3. Using the particular instrument SOP, the trainee should carry out a viscosity measurement on a suitable sample.

OTHER ANALYTICAL TECHNIQUES

DISINTEGRATION

The disintegration test is a measure of the time required under a given set of conditions for a group of tablets to disintegrate into particles.

The disintegration test is carried out using the disintegration tester. This apparatus is composed of a basket rack with six plastic tubes, open at the top and bottom, the bottom of the tube is covered by a 10-mesh screen. The basket is immersed in a 1 L beaker of suitable liquid held at 37°C.

For compressed uncoated tablets, the testing fluid is usually water at 37°C, but some monographs direct that simulated gastric fluid be used.

1. Explain the term "Disintegration" and its importance within the pharmaceutical industry.
2. Using the relevant SOP, explain how the particular disintegration apparatus works and how it is operated.
3. Attention should be drawn to take care of the sample tubes and discs.
4. Emphasize the importance of carrying out the determination at the specified temperature and by using fresh media for all determinations.

YOUR COMPANY NAME

Name: _____ ID No.: _____ Issued by: _____

Designation: _____ Department: _____ Date: _____

5. Explain the different types of coating employed—that is, enteric/non-enteric-coated tablets and show how the disintegration apparatus is used for each type of tablet.
6. Explain the difference between tablet/capsule disintegration and show that complete disintegration occurs even if coating/capsule fragments are still visible.
7. The trainee should carry out a suitable disintegration exercise.

QCT-04

Assessment of Training

QCT-04.1

Assessment Procedure for Chemical Testing

YOUR COMPANY NAME

Name: _____ ID No.: _____ Issued by: _____

Designation: _____ Department: _____ Date: _____

PROCEDURE

1. The assessment procedure will be given to the chemist under training.
2. The trainer will discuss with each analyst in a group or separately the contents of SOP No. ABC-000, which covers the keynotes regarding training aspects to be considered for the testing of chemist.
3. Each chemist will be responsible to keep his/her records updated and make entries on Annexure 1 given in SOP No. ABC-xxx.
4. Training.

USE OF BALANCE AND VOLUMETRIC TECHNIQUES

Weigh accurately a clean, dry 150 mL beaker. Add 10 mL water from 10 mL cylinder and reweigh. Calculate the volume of water added from volume = weight of water, where w = wt per mL of water at the RT.

Repeat the exercise for

10 mL water measured from a 10 mL graduated pipette
10 mL water measured from 50 mL burette
3×10 mL water measured from 10 mL Grade A pipette

Assessment—The results obtained for the 3×10 mL pipettings from the Grade A pipette should have maximum spread of 0.02 mL and the mean of three should be 10.00 + 0.02 mL.

TITRATION WITH 1.0 M HYDROCHLORIC ACID

Reagents: 1.0 M hydrochloric acid (use prepared volumetric solution); 1.0 M NaOH (use prepared volumetric solution); 0.1% phenolphthalein in 95% EtOH.

YOUR COMPANY NAME

Name: _____ ID No.: _____ Issued by: _____

Designation: _____ Department: _____ Date: _____

Procedure: Pipette 20 mL of 1.0 M NaOH into each of the three dry conical flasks. Add 1 mL of phenolphthalein into each flask and titrate with 1.0 M HCl from the burette to a colourless end point.

Criteria for acceptance: The factors obtained should have a spread of not more than 0.002 and the average of the three factors should not differ from the trainee's results by more than 0.005 f = 20.0 × 1.0 v = volume added from burette.

QUANTITATIVE TRANSFER OF SODIUM HYDROXIDE

Reagents: 1.0 M sodium hydroxide (volumetric solution); phenolphthalein solution 1% B.P; 1.0 M hydrochloric acid (volumetric solution).

Procedure: Measure from a burette, 40.0 mL 1.0 M sodium hydroxide into a 250 mL beaker. Transfer quantitatively into a 250 mL conical flask washing in with 3 × 25 mL portions of water. Add 1 mL phenolphthalein to the beaker, swirl and then transfer to the flask. Titrate with 1.0 M hydrochloric acid until colourless.

Calculation: Calculate the volume of alkali transferred,

$$s = \frac{V \times f1}{f2}$$

where

s = volume transferred
V = volume acid required
$f1$ = factor acid
$f2$ = factor alkali

Criteria for acceptance: No pink colour should be produced in the beaker. The volume of alkali transferred should be 40 + 0.05 mL.

TEMPERATURE MEASUREMENT AND CONTROL

1. The trainee should be able to use correctly, according to relevant SOPs all forms of heating and cooling used within the laboratory, that is, burners, ovens, steam or water baths, ice baths, and so on.
2. The trainee should carry out at least two determinations of the melting point or melting range of substances readily reduced to a powder according to appropriate methods.

YOUR COMPANY NAME

Name: _____ ID No.: _____ Issued by: _____

Designation: _____ Department: _____ Date: _____

Criteria for acceptance: The trainee should demonstrate appropriate and correct use of the apparatus mentioned in the sections above. The melting points or ranges obtained by the trainee should be as expected. If the trainee's results are not as expected, the trainer has to decide whether the test needs to be repeated, if necessary, after a certain period of training.

SOLVENT EXTRACTION EXERCISE

1. The trainee should carry out a routine solvent extraction exercise that is in use in the laboratory. This may take the form of either an acidic or basic precipitation, extraction of solvent, titration and so on.
2. The determination should be carried out in triplicate and the trainee's results compared with those of an experienced analyst carried out on the same sample.

Criteria for acceptance: The spread of the three results should not exceed 4.0% relative to the result and the mean of the three results should be within 2.0% of the result obtained by an experienced analyst on the same sample. The trainer has to decide whether the trainee needs to repeat the exercise, if necessary, after a certain period of training.

EXERCISE FOR LIMIT TESTS

CHLORIDE LIMIT TEST

1. The trainee should prepare two standards as given in the appropriate pharmacopoeia.
2. Carry out the test on samples or a solution containing known amount of ion (supplied by trainer) and on at least one previously tested suitable sample.

Criteria for acceptance: The two standards prepared should be virtually identical as regards to clarity and the amount of chloride found in the solution and the samples should be as expected. If the trainee's results are not within these requirements, the trainer has to decide whether the exercise needs to be repeated, if necessary, after a certain period of training.

SULPHATE LIMIT TEST

1. The trainee should prepare standards and determine the sulphate content of a supplied solution or samples.

YOUR COMPANY NAME

Name: _____ ID No.: _____ Issued by: _____

Designation: _____ Department: _____ Date: _____

2. Carry out test on samples or a solution containing known amount of ion (supplied by trainer) and on at least one previously tested suitable sample.

Criteria for acceptance: As given for the chloride limit test.

IRON LIMIT TEST

1. The trainee should prepare standards and determine the iron content of a supplied solution and samples as discussed for chloride and sulphate ions in the sections above.

Criteria for acceptance: As outlined in the sections above.

LIMIT TEST FOR LEAD OR HEAVY METALS

1. The trainee should prepare standards and determine the lead or heavy metal content of a supplied solution samples as in the sections above.

Criteria for acceptance: As given for the chloride limit test.

LIMIT TEST FOR ASH OR SULPHATED ASH

1. The trainee should carry out at least one sulphated ash determination on previously examined samples.

Criteria for acceptance: The determination should have been carried out correctly according to the appropriate specification. The results obtained should be as expected. If the trainee's results are not within these requirements, the trainer has to decide whether the exercise needs to be repeated, if necessary, after a certain period of training.

LIMIT TEST FOR LOSS ON DRYING

1. Trainee should carry out two determinations (in duplicate) on suitable previously examined samples, one of which should be hygroscopic when dry. For example, sodium carbonate, and so on.

Criteria for acceptance: The trainee must demonstrate the determinations according to the appropriate specification and the results obtained should be as expected. If the results are not within these requirements, the tests have to be repeated, if necessary, after some further training.

YOUR COMPANY NAME

Name: _____ ID No.: _____ Issued by: _____

Designation: _____ Department: _____ Date: _____

DETERMINATION OF WEIGHT PER ML AND DENSITY OF SOLID

1. The trainee should determine the weight per mL of a suitable, previously examined liquid and, if required, the apparent density of a suitable powder.

Criteria of acceptance: The determination must be carried out according to the specification and the results obtained should be as expected. If the trainee's results are not within these requirements, the trainer has to decide whether the tests need to be repeated, if necessary, after a certain period of training.

PHYSICAL OBSERVATION

1. The trainee should report the appearance, odour and solution characteristics of several suitable samples.

Criteria for acceptance: The results obtained should be as expected.

TESTING TO SPECIFICATION/PRACTICAL WORK

1. An experienced analyst should have previously tested the practical work or samples tested by the trainee.
2. In all cases, the results obtained by the trainee should be within the accuracy and precision of the methods carried out and similar to those obtained by an experienced analyst.

Criteria for acceptance: If the trainee's results do not meet these requirements, the trainer has to decide whether the tests have to be repeated and, if necessary, carry out further training as required.

The trainee should not be allowed to carry out actual work until the trainer is satisfied that he/she has reached an acceptable standard.

CHROMATOGRAPHIC TECHNIQUES

Assessment procedure for TLC:

1. The trainee should first carry out a simple routine TLC method, currently in use within the laboratory, following the normal specification.

YOUR COMPANY NAME

Name: _____ ID No.: _____ Issued by: _____

Designation: _____ Department: _____ Date: _____

2. The trainer should then assess the following:
   a. The chromatographic plate has been marked correctly.
   b. The chromatographic plate has been developed correctly.
   c. The chromatographic plate is free from fingerprints and spurious spots.
   d. The Rf values of the spots are correct.
   e. The intensities of the spots are as expected.
   f. The data are recorded correctly in notebooks and/or on photographs.
   g. The trainee should then assess the relative intensities of a series of spots of different loadings, spotted in random order.
   h. This plate should be prepared and developed in advance by the trainer with six spots applied with loadings in proportion 1:2:3:4:5:6.

Criteria for acceptance:

a. The TLC should be carried out according to the principles given ensuring correct marking, development and recording of data.
b. The assessment of the intensities of the spots on given chromatogram should be in the correct order.
c. If the trainee's results are not within these requirements, the training should be repeated, if necessary, after a certain period of training.

ASSESSMENT PROCEDURES FOR GC AND HPLC

Outline procedures are given below to form the basis of assessment tests for trainees in the techniques of HPLC and GC. These procedures are independent of the actual equipment used, and require only the essential basic components of a GC or HPLC system, although more sophisticated equipment may of course be utilized. The set-up and operational details of each particular GC or HPLC system are not included in these procedures, and the assessment is thus not instrument specific but provides a test of the trainee's ability to carry out an analysis using these techniques. Similarly, the use of internal and external standardization (or both) can be tested as desired using these same basic procedures. Typically, external standardization may be used in HPLC with a fixed-loop injection valve, or in GC analysis for residue determinations, whereas internal standardization may be used in HPLC or GC analysis where injection volume is controlled by a microlitre syringe. The actual analytical method used can be selected to suit the work of each section or department. However, it should be an

YOUR COMPANY NAME

Name: _____ ID No.: _____ Issued by: _____

Designation: _____ Department: _____ Date: _____

established, reliable method, and should involve the minimum of sample preparation (as it is the chromatographic analysis which is to be assessed). For a residue method, it may even be preferable to provide a test solution rather than original sample.

Once selected, a copy of the method should be given to the trainee so that the trainee has sufficient information to prepare the solutions and run the chromatographic analysis. The sample (or test solution), which the trainee is required to analyse, should be a known one, previously analysed by practicing and competent analyst.

TEST PROCEDURE

CHROMATOGRAPHIC APPARATUS

1. As indicated above, only the essential components of a chromatographic system are required for these procedures, but the actual system used may vary from very basic manual instruments to sophisticated automated instruments.
2. The trainee should not be expected, as a part of this test, to be fully conversant with all operational details of each piece of equipment. The supervising analyst should in fact ensure that the equipment is in proper working order and show the trainee how to work it at a level, which permits the assessment test to be performed properly.
3. For HPLC systems:
   a. An isocratic method is recommended in order to avoid unnecessary complications.
   b. The type of injection system used is optional, but is recommended that external standardization be tested only if a fixed loop injection valve is used.
   c. A UV detector will be assumed.
   d. Peak measurement may be electronic measurement of area (or height) or manual measurement of height.
4. For GC systems:
   a. An isothermal method is recommended in order to avoid unnecessary complications.
   b. It is worthwhile to adopt manual injection (rather than use of an auto-injector) in order to include in the overall test, the trainee's ability to manipulate a microlitre syringe and inject via a septum.

YOUR COMPANY NAME

Name: _____ ID No.: _____ Issued by: _____

Designation: _____ Department: _____ Date: _____

    c. The type of oven, nature of carrier gas, and so on, need not be fixed, and it is useful in a GC assessment to accommodate the use of any desired type of detector, for example, FID, TCD.

    d. Peak measurement may be electronic or manual as in the section above for HPLC.

EQUIPMENT PREPARATION

5. The supervising analyst should guide the trainee in selecting and fitting the required column, initializing gas and power supplies to the equipment, and entering the required operational parameters at the chromatograph, detector and integrator.

6. For HPLC, the trainee should prepare and degas the mobile phase according to the details given in the analytical method, and the pump mobile phase at required flow rate and allow the column to equilibrate and establish a stable baseline.

7. For GC, once gas flows to column and detector have been correctly adjusted and injector, column and detector temperature set, the system should then be allowed to equilibrate and establish a stable baseline.

Finally, the supervisor should demonstrate the operation of the equipment, that is, how to make an injection run the chromatogram and collect the data.

PREPARATION OF SOLUTIONS

8. The trainee should prepare standard and sample solutions according to details given in the particular analytical method being used.

9. This method will specify whether or not to add internal standard.

10. For residue method, a test solution may be provided obviating the need for preparing a sample solution.

CHROMATOGRAPHY

11. Using the solution prepared in the sections above and the operating conditions set-up (both obtained from the analytical method), the trainee should carry out the following:

    a. Chromatograph the standard solution twice and ignore these runs.

    b. Chromatograph the standard solution three times and measure the peaks in each case.

YOUR COMPANY NAME

Name: _____ ID No.: _____ Issued by: _____

Designation: _____ Department: _____ Date: _____

    c. Chromatograph the sample solution twice and measure the peaks in each case.
    d. Chromatograph the standard solution once more and measure the peaks.

CALCULATION OF RESULTS

12. If internal standardization is specified in the method, the trainee should calculate the peak area (or height) ratio of test compound to internal standard on each of the six chromatograms run.
13. Using the peak ratios (for internal standardization) or otherwise the actual peak heights or areas for the test compound, the trainee should then
    a. Calculate the mean, relative standard deviation and maximum spread (largest result, smallest result) as percentage of mean, for the first three standards.
    b. Calculate the mean of the two samples, and the mean of the two standards adjacent to the samples, and use their values to calculate the sample result as follows:

$$\text{Test compound in sample, } \% \text{ w/w} = \frac{S \times Wr \times P \times F}{R \times Ws}$$

where S is the mean peak ratio (compound: IS) or peak area/height from duplicate standard chromatograms; Wr is the weight ratio (compound: IS), or weight of standard compound, in standard solution; Ws is the weight ratio (sample: IS), or weight of sample, in sample solution; P is the % purity of compound standard; F is the any dilution factor required.

    This calculation may be modified in the case where a test solution was provided: in any case, details may be obtained either from the analytical method or from the supervising analyst.

CRITERIA FOR ASSESSMENT

1. *Chromatographic precision:* For the three standards, the maximum spread, expressed as % of the mean, should be within the tolerance quoted in the analytical method and the relative standard deviation

YOUR COMPANY NAME

Name: _____ ID No.: _____ Issued by: _____

Designation: _____ Department: _____ Date: _____

should be within the limits set by experienced analysts familiar with the
method.

2. *Accuracy:* The trainee's result for the sample should be judged against
   the result obtained by the experienced analyst on the same sample by the
   same method. Agreement should be within the accuracy tolerance quoted
   in the analytical method.

3. *Comments:* The precision and accuracy attainable will depend on the
   analytical methods used for the assessment test, but as a guide the following values are typical.

QCT-04.2

Assessment Procedure
for Microbiologist

YOUR COMPANY NAME

Name: _____ ID No.: _____ Issued by: _____

Designation: _____ Department: _____ Date: _____

PROCEDURE

The trainer and the trainee will be responsible to keep the training log updated.

USE OF BALANCE AND VOLUMETRIC TECHNIQUES

Weight accurately a clean, weighing bottle. Add 10 mL water from a 10 mL cylinder and reweigh. Calculate the volume of water added from volume = weight of water, where w = wt mL of water at the RT.

REPEAT THE EXERCISE

10 mL water measured from a 50 mL cylinder
10 mL water measured from a 10 mL graduated pipette
10 mL water measured form a 50 mL burette
3 × 10 mL water measured from a 10 mL one mark pipette of known calibration

ASSESSMENT

The results obtained for the 3 × 10 mL pipettings from the one mark pipette should have a maximum spread of 0.02 mL and the mean of the three should be 10.00 + 0.02 mL.

TEMPERATURE MEASUREMENT AND CONTROL

1. The trainee should be able to use correctly, according to relevant SOPs, all forms of heating and cooling used within the laboratory—that is, burners, ovens, steam or water baths, ice baths, and so on.

YOUR COMPANY NAME

Name: _____ ID No.: _____ Issued by: _____

Designation: _____ Department: _____ Date: _____

2. The trainee should carry out at least two determinations of the melting point or melting range of substance readily reduced to a powder according to appropriate methods.

Criteria for acceptance: The trainee should have used the apparatus, and so on covered in Section 2.1 correctly. The melting points or ranges obtained by the trainee should be as expected. If the trainee's results are not as expected, the trainer has to decide whether the tests need to be repeated, if necessary, after a certain period of training.

MEDIA PREPARATION

1. The trainee should prepare any two types of liquid media and any two types of solid media.

Criteria for acceptance: The appearance, that is, colour, clarity and solidification, if appropriate, should all be as given in the manufacturer's guidelines.

The appropriate organism(s) should be cultured on/in the media and growth and appearance should be as in the manufacturer's guidelines.

GLASSWARE PREPARATION

The trainee should spend at least a week preparing and washing all forms of glassware.

ASEPTIC TECHNIQUE

The acceptability of the trainee's technique will become apparent during the normal days as controls are used in various tests to check for contamination and aseptic procedures.

AUTOCLAVES

The trainee should carry out calibration of the autoclaves in accordance with instructions in the operating manual and corresponding SOPs.

Criteria for acceptance: Providing the autoclave is functioning properly, all calibration checks should be in accordance with instructions in the operating manual and corresponding SOPs.

YOUR COMPANY NAME

Name: _____ ID No.: _____ Issued by: _____

Designation: _____ Department: _____ Date: _____

TESTING TO SPECIFICATION/PRACTICAL WORK

1. An experienced analyst should test the practical work or samples tested by the trainee.
2. In all cases, the results obtained by the trainee should be within the accuracy and precision of the methods carried out and similar to those obtained by an experienced analyst.
3. If the trainee's results do not meet the requirements, the trainer has to decide whether any test(s) needs repeating and, if necessary, carry out further training.
4. The trainee should not be allowed to carry out actual work until the trainer is satisfied that he/she has reached an acceptable standard.

MICROBIOLOGICAL ASSAYS

1. The trainee should first carry out an assay using approved method.
2. The trainer should assess the following:
    a. Assay plates or trays have been marked correctly.
    b. The required information has been entered into appropriate books and that the computer printouts also have this information.
    c. Accuracy of assay is compared to previous assay on the same lot of product.
    d. All check samples, if necessary, are within limits.
    e. The raw data are within the acceptable limits so as to give appropriate valid assays.

Criteria for acceptance:

1. The assay has been carried out in accordance with the principles given in the STM and appropriate SOP, ensuring correct marking and identification of assay plates and trays.
2. The assay is in the required range of previous assays and the check samples are within the required control limits.
3. If the trainee's results are not within these requirements, the trainer has to decide whether the exercise should be repeated, if necessary, after a certain period of training.

YOUR COMPANY NAME

Name: _____ ID No.: _____ Issued by: _____

Designation: _____ Department: _____ Date: _____

pH MEASUREMENT

1. The trainee should prepare a suitable solution and measure its pH according to the relevant SOP.
2. An experienced analyst should have previously analysed all samples used.

Criteria for acceptance:

1. The trainee should carry out the procedures according to the appropriate method and corresponding SOP and the results obtained should be as expected.
2. If these requirements are not met, the trainer has to decide whether the tests need to be repeated, if necessary, after a certain period of training.

ENVIRONMENTAL MONITORING

The trainee should carry out appropriate air sampling and water sampling techniques in conjunction with the trainer.

Criteria of acceptance: The results, that is, the number of organism determined by the trainer and the trainee should be similar.

AEROBIC MICROBIAL COUNTS ORGANISM IDENTIFICATION

1. *Salmonella*, *Escherichia coli*, *Pseudomonas* and *Staphylococcus* all have positive control tests, which need to be carried out at some stage.
2. The trainee, when conversant with GLP and aseptic techniques, should carry out these positive controls.
3. For the microbial counts, an unknown quantity of organism will be assigned to the trainee, which should be tested as necessary.
4. The trainer will also carry out AMC on the same sample to determine the number of organisms present.

Criteria for acceptance:

1. The positive controls should be carried out with GLP and acceptable aseptic technique and the trainee should isolate all the relevant organisms.
2. It should also be noted here that identification of organisms is necessary and the trainee would be expected to carry out that function as well.

YOUR COMPANY NAME

Name: _____ ID No.: _____ Issued by: _____

Designation: _____ Department: _____ Date: _____

MAINTENANCE OF CULTURES AND ORGANISM IDENTIFICATION

The trainee will be supplied with a range of organisms to which he will be expected to give a name.

Criteria of acceptance: Other analytical techniques:

1. Where possible, assessment procedures should be devised and implemented for other important techniques in use in the laboratory.
2. In all cases, the trainee's accuracy and precision should be compared with that obtained by an experienced analyst.
3. An experienced analyst should have previously examined the practical work or testing to specification given to the trainees.

QCT-05

Training Assessment with Quiz and Answers

QCT-05.1

Assessment for Analytical Methods Validation and Requirements

YOUR COMPANY NAME

Name: _____ ID No.: _____ Issued by: _____

Designation: _____ Department: _____ Date: _____

Fill in the blanks using appropriate words from the given multiple choices.

1. Analytical methods validation is a gauge taken to prove that the analytical methods employed for a specific test will produce results that consistently meet _____ specifications.
   a. In-process
   b. Final products
   c. Predetermined
   d. Raw material

2. The products quality is very much based on the _____, change control, validation and training of the analytical testing methods.
   a. Documentation
   b. Specifications
   c. Development
   d. Batch audit

3. All the quality standards used by the laboratory should be complying with the _____ monograph requirements.
   a. United States Pharmacopeia
   b. British Pharmacopoeia
   c. European Pharmacopoeia
   d. USP, BP and EP

YOUR COMPANY NAME

Name: _____ ID No.: _____ Issued by: _____

Designation: _____ Department: _____ Date: _____

4. A test method _____ must be in place supported by a general SOP or method validation protocol for each product.
   a. Procedure
   b. Document
   c. Validation master plan
   d. All of above

5. "Limit of Detection" and "Limit of Quantitation" are tests to be included in the _____ for a test method validation.
   a. Master validation plan
   b. Validation protocol
   c. Standard test method
   d. Change control request

6. Any change in the analytical method validation protocol must seek authorization by _____.
   a. Research and development
   b. Quality control laboratory
   c. Quality assurance
   d. Production control

7. A written procedure needs to be available which prohibits making any changes except those _____ by QA.
   a. Authorized
   b. Requested
   c. Prohibited
   d. Initiated

8. Changes in laboratory analytical methods may impact product quality and _____.
   a. Product release criteria
   b. Regulatory commitments
   c. Product specifications
   d. Product stability

YOUR COMPANY NAME

Name: _____ ID No.: _____ Issued by: _____

Designation: _____ Department: _____ Date: _____

9. All changes in test methods are governed by a _____, according to which the proposals, evaluation and implementation of changes could be controlled.
   a. Method
   b. System
   c. Person
   d. Protocol

10. The change control system requires that a changed method be _____ prior to implementation of the change and release of product using the method.
    a. Transferred
    b. Re-validated
    c. Executed
    d. Verified

11. The QSMs must always be in the _____.
    a. Current revision state
    b. Laboratory's cupboard
    c. Appropriate file
    d. Manager's office only

12. A periodic verification/reconciliation must be carried out to ensure the current status of all _____.
    a. Specifications
    b. Quality standards manuals
    c. Standard operating procedures
    d. a and c

13. Training files for laboratory analysts must contain the following information:
    a. SOP training documentation
    b. Analytical methods/quality manuals training
    c. Analytical instrument training
    d. a, b and c

YOUR COMPANY NAME

Name: _____ ID No.: _____ Issued by: _____

Designation: _____ Department: _____ Date: _____

14. All _____ and test results will be recorded in bound and pre-numbered workbooks.
    a. Calculations
    b. Raw data
    c. Product details
    d. Analytical

15. The raw data check system must include a careful examination of _____ and _____ as a minimum.
    a. Weighing
    b. Dilutions
    c. Product's strength
    d. Expiry date of product

16. Vendor's _____ must be kept on file with other data, and accessible for review for each raw material.
    a. History and background
    b. Audit report
    c. Certificate of analysis
    d. Stability report

17. In case QC lab has a reduced testing program in place then a _____ is required to be available to describe as to when reduced testing can be instituted.
    a. Standard operating procedure
    b. Validation protocol
    c. Master plan
    d. Quality assurance approval

QCT-05.1.1

Answers to Quiz for Analytical Methods Validation and Requirements

YOUR COMPANY NAME

Name: _____ ID No.: _____ Issued by: _____

Designation: _____ Department: _____ Date: _____

1. Analytical methods validation is a gauge taken to prove that the analytical methods employed for a specific test will produce results that consistently meet _____ specifications.
   Predetermined

2. The products quality is very much based on the _____, change control, validation and training of the analytical testing methods.
   Documentation

3. All the quality standards used by the laboratory should be complying with the _____ monograph requirements.
   USP, BP and EP

4. A test method _____ must be in place supported by a general SOP or method validation protocol for each product.
   Validation master plan

5. "Limit of Detection" and "Limit of Quantitation" are tests to be included in the _____ for a test method validation.
   Validation protocol

6. Any change in the analytical method validation protocol must seek authorization by _____.
   Quality assurance

YOUR COMPANY NAME

Name: _____ ID No.: _____ Issued by: _____

Designation: _____ Department: _____ Date: _____

7. A written procedure needs to be available which prohibits making any changes except those _____ by QA.
   Authorized

8. Changes in laboratory analytical methods may impact product quality and _____.
   Regulatory commitments

9. All changes in test methods are governed by a _____ according to which the proposals, evaluation and implementation of changes could be controlled.
   System

10. The change control system requires that a changed method be _____ prior to implementation of the change and release of product using the method.
    Revalidated

11. The QSMs must always be in the _____.
    Current revision state

12. A periodic verification/reconciliation must be carried out to ensure the current status of all _____.
    Quality standards manuals

13. Training files for laboratory analysts must contain the following information:
    a, b and c

14. All _____ and test results will be recorded in bound and pre-numbered workbooks.
    Raw data

15. The raw data check system must include a careful examination of _____ and _____ as a minimum.
    Weighing and dilutions

16. Vendor's _____ must be kept on file with other data, and accessible for review for each raw material.
    Certificate of analysis

YOUR COMPANY NAME

Name: _____ ID No.: _____ Issued by: _____

Designation: _____ Department: _____ Date: _____

17. In case QC lab has a reduced testing programme in place then a _____ is required to be available to describe as to when reduced testing can be instituted.
    Standard operating procedure

QCT-05.2

Assessment for Analytical Equipment

YOUR COMPANY NAME

Name: _____ ID No.: _____ Issued by: _____

Designation: _____ Department: _____ Date: _____

1. The _____ and _____ of the analytical instrument play a vital role in pharmaceutical industry to obtain valid data.
   a. Model and make
   b. Accuracy and precision
   c. Cleaning and maintenance
   d. Handling and calibration

2. Companies are required to establish _____ assuring that the users of analytical instruments are trained to perform their assigned tasks.
   a. Experts
   b. Procedures
   c. Reports
   d. Plans

3. The advent of _____, calibration and preventive maintenance activities allows laboratory equipment to continuously operate within operating parameters.
   a. Qualification
   b. Standard operating procedures
   c. Automated systems
   d. GLP

4. Calibration, maintenance, cleaning, change control and qualification of laboratory instruments must be addressed in _____.
   a. Site master plan
   b. Site policies and procedures
   c. Quality manual
   d. Validation protocol

YOUR COMPANY NAME

Name: _____ ID No.: _____ Issued by: _____

Designation: _____ Department: _____ Date: _____

5. Mechanism for assigning tolerances and frequencies should be a part of the _____.
   a. Master validation plan
   b. Calibration program
   c. Standard operating procedure
   d. Instruments logbook

6. The QC laboratory or the maintenance department should have _____, which includes all pieces of laboratory equipment that needed routine calibration.
   a. Instrument manual
   b. Inventory logbook
   c. Master instrument list
   d. Master calibration list

7. Procedure for calibration of analytical instruments should contain the following except _____.
   a. Schedule for calibration
   b. Responsible persons for calibration
   c. Calibration tolerances
   d. Analyst's training

8. The calibration standards for each piece of laboratory instrument must be traceable to the _____.
   a. Calibration master plan
   b. Master standard
   c. Preventive plan
   d. Calibration record

9. Frequent checks of the _____ must be performed to ensure that worksheets and electronic printouts generated from laboratory equipment are complete and accurate.
   a. Analyst's workbook
   b. Instruments logbook
   c. Instruments manual
   d. Calibration record

YOUR COMPANY NAME

Name: _____ ID No.: _____ Issued by: _____

Designation: _____ Department: _____ Date: _____

10. Procedure for dismantling and reassembling of equipment where necessary to assure proper cleaning, must be part of _____.
    a. Equipment master validation plan
    b. Maintenance and preventive SOP
    c. Cleaning and sanitization SOP
    d. Calibration plan

11. Companies must ensure availability of _____ to address qualification of analytical instruments and equipment.
    a. Validation protocol
    b. Written procedure
    c. Master plan
    d. GMP guidelines

12. None of the analytical instrument could be used without _____.
    a. Qualification
    b. Handling manual
    c. Validation protocol
    d. Standard test methods

13. There must be a system in place, which may prevent the use of the _____.
    a. Unclean equipment
    b. Old equipment
    c. Non-qualified equipment
    d. New equipment

14. All HPLC units will be _____ every year or as per the frequency established in the SOP.
    a. Cleaned and sanitized
    b. Dismantled and reassembled
    c. Re-qualified
    d. Calibrated

YOUR COMPANY NAME

Name: _____ ID No.: _____ Issued by: _____

Designation: _____ Department: _____ Date: _____

15. The general SOP for IQ, OQ, and PQ must also describe in detail the requirement of _____ prior to commencing the qualification process.
    a. Master plan
    b. Approved protocol
    c. GMP guidelines
    d. Permission of QA

16. _____ test must also be carried out during the annual re-qualification of a pump associated with an HPLC unit.
    a. Linearity
    b. Carryover
    c. Wavelength accuracy
    d. Composition accuracy

17. A written procedure must be established to describe the steps and measures taken for maintaining HPLC and GLC _____ inventory.
    a. Columns
    b. Detectors
    c. Standards
    d. Mobile phase

18. The _____ with the column number on it will be filed in the respective data binder.
    a. Test chromatogram
    b. Box
    c. Receipt
    d. Purchase order

19. Changes to the calibration standards and frequencies shall be governed by a _____ procedure.
    a. Change control
    b. Calibration
    c. Validation
    d. Maintenance master plan

YOUR COMPANY NAME

Name: _____ ID No.: _____ Issued by: _____

Designation: _____ Department: _____ Date: _____

20. When the column is finally _____, the reason must be recorded in the logbook.
    a. Qualified
    b. Changed
    c. Discarded
    d. Used

QCT-05.2.1

Answers to Quiz for Analytical Equipment

YOUR COMPANY NAME

Name: _____ ID No.: _____ Issued by: _____

Designation: _____ Department: _____ Date: _____

1. The _____ and _____ of the analytical instrument play a vital role in pharmaceutical industry to obtain valid data.
   Accuracy and precision

2. Companies are required to establish _____ assuring that the users of analytical instruments are trained to perform their assigned tasks.
   Procedures

3. The advent of _____, calibration and preventive maintenance activities allows for laboratory equipment to continuously operate within operating parameters.
   Qualification

4. Calibration, maintenance, cleaning, change control and qualification of laboratory instruments must be addressed in _____.
   Site policies and procedures

5. Mechanism for assigning tolerances and frequencies should be a part of the _____.
   Standard operating procedure

6. The QC laboratory or the maintenance department should have _____, which includes all pieces of laboratory equipment that needed routine calibration.
   Master calibration list

YOUR COMPANY NAME

Name: _____ ID No.: _____ Issued by: _____

Designation: _____ Department: _____ Date: _____

7. The procedure for calibration of analytical instruments should contain the following except _____.
   Analyst's training

8. The calibration standards for each piece of laboratory instrument must be traceable to the _____.
   Master standard

9. Frequent checks of the _____ must be performed to ensure that worksheets and electronic printouts generated from laboratory equipment are complete and accurate.
   Instruments logbook

10. Procedure for dismantling and reassembling of equipment where necessary to assure proper cleaning, must be part of _____.
    Cleaning and sanitization SOP

11. Companies must ensure availability of _____ to address qualification of analytical instruments and equipment.
    Written procedure

12. None of the analytical instrument could be used without _____.
    Qualification

13. There must be a system in place, which may prevent the use of the _____.
    Non-qualified equipment

14. All HPLC units will be _____ every year or as per the frequency established in the SOP.
    Re-qualified

15. The general SOP for IQ, OQ, and PQ must also describe in detail the requirement of _____ prior to commencing the qualification process.
    Approved protocol

YOUR COMPANY NAME

Name: _____ ID No.: _____ Issued by: _____

Designation: _____ Department: _____ Date: _____

16. _____ test must also be carried out during the annual re-qualification of a pump associated with an HPLC unit.
Composition accuracy

17. A written procedure must be established to describe the steps and measures taken for maintaining HPLC and GLC _____ inventory.
Columns

18. The _____ with the column number on it will be filed in the respective data binder.
Test chromatogram

19. Change to the calibration standards and frequencies shall be governed by a _____ procedure.
Change control

20. When the column is finally _____, the reason must be recorded in the logbook.
Discarded

QCT-05.3

Assessment for Reference Standards and Reagents

YOUR COMPANY NAME

Name: _____ ID No.: _____ Issued by: _____

Designation: _____ Department: _____ Date: _____

1. Ordering and receipt of USP and other compendial reference standards must be done as per _____.
   a. Purchase order
   b. Written procedure
   c. Requirement
   d. Site policy

2. All reagents are _____ with the date of receipt, the date the bottle is opened and the initials of the person opening.
   a. Kept
   b. Labelled
   c. Purchased
   d. Registered

3. Availability of correct lot number of all pharmacopoeia standards can be ensured by routine review of the corresponding _____.
   a. SOP
   b. Raw material specifications
   c. Pharmacopoeia forum
   d. Material logbook

4. The written procedure must also outline the need of periodical inventory check and documentation in a logbook to assure that only _____ are in use.
   a. 100% pure standards
   b. Current lots
   c. Primary standards
   d. Correct standards

YOUR COMPANY NAME

Name: _____ ID No.: _____ Issued by: _____

Designation: _____ Department: _____ Date: _____

5. Out of date lots must be _____.
   a. Re-standardized
   b. Stored in the reference samples room
   c. Kept in a cool and dry place
   d. Destroyed

6. All primary reference standards must be stored under the _____.
   a. Recommended storage conditions
   b. Lock and key
   c. Supervision of manager
   d. Cold atmosphere

7. The standards storage location should be secured in to which access is limited only to laboratory personnel having a _____.
   a. Experience certificate
   b. Permission letter
   c. Management authority
   d. Logbook

8. A mechanism needs to be established in the laboratory for ensuring that _____ reagents are not used.
   a. Expired
   b. Old
   c. Same
   d. Critical

9. To keep a better control over the usage of reagents within valid dates, analysts must record the _____ and expiry date of the reagents while conducting a particular test.
   a. Lot number
   b. Supplier's name
   c. Receiving date
   d. Standardization date

YOUR COMPANY NAME

Name: _____ ID No.: _____ Issued by: _____

Designation: _____ Department: _____ Date: _____

10. The test for _____ could be used to assure reagent identification and integrity throughout expiry and use.
    a. Moisture
    b. Purity and potency
    c. Concentration
    d. Physical attributes

11. After the material is identified as a potential internal working standard, testing for _____ is performed.
    a. Characterization
    b. Potency
    c. Identification
    d. Standardization

12. The intermediate container and packaging components of the material must be _____ at the time of receipt.
    a. Dated
    b. Marked
    c. Intact and in good conditions
    d. Named properly

13. Reference standard samples must be taken under _____ into clean, dry, sterilized containers of adequate size and provided with hermetic seal.
    a. Laminar flow conditions
    b. Appropriate temperature
    c. Manager's supervision
    d. Lock and key

14. A total of _____ tests per sample will be performed to determine the potency of each sample.
    a. Six
    b. Three
    c. Nine
    d. One

YOUR COMPANY NAME

Name: _____ ID No.: _____ Issued by: _____

Designation: _____ Department: _____ Date: _____

15. The samples of materials for _____ as internal working stan-
    dards will be tested against current GMP standards.
    a. Identification
    b. Qualification
    c. Analysis
    d. Reference

16. A system should be in place to verify that standards, reagents or solution
    are _____ prior to their use.
    a. Available
    b. Ordered
    c. In date
    d. Purchased

17. The SOP should clearly state how many times as a maximum number
    the flask might be opened before the stock solution must be
    _____.
    a. Discarded
    b. Re-qualified
    c. Analysed
    d. Released for use

18. The traceability of the _____ of standards, reagents or solution
    used for a particular test must also be ensured through a mechanism.
    a. Lot number
    b. Expiration date
    c. Preparation date
    d. Manufacturer

19. Storage of stock solution, reagents and standards should be done in a
    manner, which prevents _____ or degradation.
    a. Breakage
    b. Contamination
    c. Oxidation
    d. Lost

YOUR COMPANY NAME

Name: _____ ID No.: _____ Issued by: _____

Designation: _____ Department: _____ Date: _____

20. Storage conditions must also be strictly maintained as recommended for each type of _____.
    a. Standards
    b. Reagents
    c. Solutions
    d. Standards, reagents, or solutions

QCT-05.3.1

Answers to Quiz for Reference Standards and Reagents

YOUR COMPANY NAME

Name: _____ ID No.: _____ Issued by: _____

Designation: _____ Department: _____ Date: _____

1. Ordering and receipt of USP and other compendial reference standards must be done as per _____.
   Written procedure

2. All reagents are _____ with the date of receipt, the date the bottle is opened and the initials of the person opening.
   Labelled

3. Availability of correct lot number of all pharmacopoeia standards can be ensured by routine review of the corresponding _____.
   Pharmacopoeia forum

4. The written procedure must also outline the need of periodical inventory check and documentation in a logbook to assure that only _____ are in use.
   Current lots

5. Outdated lots must be _____.
   Destroyed

6. All primary reference standards must be stored under the _____.
   Recommended storage conditions

YOUR COMPANY NAME

Name: _____ ID No.: _____ Issued by: _____

Designation: _____ Department: _____ Date: _____

7. The standards storage location should be secured in to which access is limited only to laboratory personnel having a _____.
Management authority

8. A mechanism needs to be established in the laboratory for ensuring that _____ reagents are not used.
Expired

9. To keep a better control over the usage of reagents within valid dates, analysts must record the _____ and expiry date of the reagents while conducting a particular test.
Lot number

10. The test for _____ could be used to assure reagent identification and integrity throughout expiry and use.
Purity and potency

11. After the material is identified as a potential internal working standard, testing for _____ is performed.
Characterization

12. The intermediate container and packaging components of the material must be _____ at the time of receipt.
Intact and in good conditions

13. Reference standard samples must be taken under _____ into clean, dry, sterilized containers of adequate size and provided with hermetic seal.
Laminar flow conditions

14. A total of _____ tests per sample will be performed to determine the potency of each sample.
Nine

15. The samples of materials for _____ as internal working standards will be tested against current GMP standards.
Qualification

YOUR COMPANY NAME

Name: _____ ID No.: _____ Issued by: _____

Designation: _____ Department: _____ Date: _____

16. A system should be in place to verify that standards, reagents or solution are _____ prior to their use.
    In date

17. The SOP should clearly state how many times as a maximum number the flask might be opened before the stock solution must be
    _____.
    Discarded

18. The traceability of the _____ of standards, reagents or solution used for a particular test must also be ensured through a mechanism.
    Expiration date

19. Storage of stock solution, reagents and standards should be done in a manner, which prevents _____ or degradation.
    Contamination

20. Storage conditions must also be strictly maintained as recommended for each type of _____.
    Standards, reagents, or solutions

QCT-05.4

Assessment for Sample Management

YOUR COMPANY NAME

Name: _____ ID No.: _____ Issued by: _____

Designation: _____ Department: _____ Date: _____

1. The results of any analysis can only be meaningful if the _____ is undertaken effectively.
   a. Processing
   b. Testing
   c. Sampling
   d. Reviewing

2. Products manufacturers need to ensure that any sample taken for analysis is _____ of the product.
   a. Derived
   b. True representative
   c. Waste material
   d. Surplus amount

3. The sampling of raw and packaging materials and their retention has to be described in a _____.
   a. Written procedure
   b. Batch document
   c. Laboratory logbook
   d. Quality assurance manual

4. A _____ must be established with scientific justification and statistical criteria such as confidence levels, component variability, degree of precision desired and the past history of supplier.
   a. Master validation plan
   b. Analytical method
   c. Sampling plan
   d. Final report

YOUR COMPANY NAME

Name: _____ ID No.: _____ Issued by: _____

Designation: _____ Department: _____ Date: _____

5. A written procedure must address exact number of samples specified for different _____ and batch size, and so on.
   a. Batches
   b. Dosage forms
   c. Products
   d. Lot numbers

6. Sampling plan should also include sample size and _____ in case of powders, granules, and liquids.
   a. Name of sampler
   b. Sample locations
   c. Type of tests to be done
   d. Name of process

7. The mount of samples taken must be sufficient for the quantity needed for analysis, retesting in case of OOS and _____.
   a. Retention sample
   b. Reserve sample
   c. Re-validation sample
   d. Stability sample

8. In case there is a change in the sampling plan, _____ must review and authorize change before implementation.
   a. Production control
   b. In-process
   c. Quality assurance
   d. Quality control

9. All activities related to sample flow including sampling, sample login, storage, assignment to analyst, testing, results documenting, retention and finally _____ should be performed as per approved procedure.
   a. Release of sample
   b. Destruction of sample
   c. Stability study of sample
   d. Validation study

YOUR COMPANY NAME

Name: _____ ID No.: _____ Issued by: _____

Designation: _____ Department: _____ Date: _____

10. Samples should always be done by _____ personnel who are not only designated to pull samples but are also appropriately trained.
    a. Senior and experienced
    b. Specific and authorized
    c. New and fresh
    d. Production

11. All sampling techniques for each specific product type must be addressed in _____.
    a. Batch document
    b. Master formula
    c. Written procedures
    d. Sampling plan

12. Procedures for cleaning of sampling tools should be _____ and included in the cleaning validation master plan except for the ones, which are dedicated or disposable.
    a. Developed
    b. Validated
    c. Written
    d. Confidential

13. Containers should be immediately re-sealed after sampling to avoid _____.
    a. Theft
    b. Mix-up
    c. Cross contamination
    d. Wastage

14. Materials which are more susceptible to contamination, should be sampled in _____ area.
    a. Open area
    b. Controlled area
    c. Cold area
    d. Quarantine area

YOUR COMPANY NAME

Name: _____ ID No.: _____ Issued by: _____

Designation: _____ Department: _____ Date: _____

15. All samples including the retention ones must be stored in containers meeting _____ and specified storage conditions.
    a. Regulatory requirements
    b. Stability requirements
    c. Quality requirements
    d. Physical parameters

16. The retention samples must be of _____ the quantity necessary for all tests required to determine that the active ingredient meets its established specifications.
    a. Thrice
    b. Twice
    c. Similar
    d. Lesser

17. All retention samples of active materials are to be retained for _____ after expiry of the last lot of the product containing the material.
    a. One year
    b. Two years
    c. Six months
    d. Five years

18. There must be a mechanism in place to assure _____ of retention samples.
    a. Safety
    b. Quality
    c. Accountability
    d. Storage

19. In case the _____ are opened and used to test for investigation, documentation must be done to indicate reason for opening to keep the track of usage.
    a. Finished products
    b. Raw materials
    c. Retention samples
    d. Packaging samples

QCT-05.4.1

Answers to Quiz for Sample Management

YOUR COMPANY NAME

Name: _____ ID No.: _____ Issued by: _____

Designation: _____ Department: _____ Date: _____

1. The results of any analysis can only be meaningful if the _____ is undertaken effectively.
   Sampling

2. Products manufacturers need to ensure that any sample taken for analysis is _____ of the product.
   True representative

3. The sampling of raw and packaging materials and their retention has to be described in a _____.
   Written procedure

4. A _____ must be established with scientific justification and statistical criteria such as confidence levels, component variability, degree of precision desired, and the past history of supplier.
   Sampling plan

5. A written procedure must address exact number of samples specified for different _____ and batch size, and so on.
   Dosage forms

6. Sampling plan should also include sample size and _____ in case of powders, granules and liquids.
   Sample locations

7. The amount of samples taken must be sufficient for the quantity needed for analysis, retesting in case of OOS and _____.
   Retention sample

YOUR COMPANY NAME

Name: _____ ID No.: _____ Issued by: _____

Designation: _____ Department: _____ Date: _____

8. In case there is a change in the sampling plan, _____ must review and authorize change before implementation.
Quality assurance

9. All activities related to sample flow including sampling, sample login, storage, assignment to analyst, testing, results documenting, retention and finally _____ should be performed as per approved procedure.
Destruction of sample

10. Samples should always be done by _____ personnel who are not only designated to pull samples but are also appropriately trained.
Specific and authorized

11. All sampling techniques for each specific product type must be addressed in _____.
Written procedures

12. Procedures for cleaning of sampling tools should be _____ and included in the cleaning validation Master plan except for the ones, which are dedicated or disposable.
Validated

13. Containers should be immediately re-sealed after sampling to avoid _____.
Cross contamination

14. Materials which are more susceptible to contamination, should be sampled in _____ area.
Controlled area

15. All samples including the retention ones must be stored in containers meeting _____ and specified storage conditions.
Regulatory requirements

16. The retention samples must be of _____ the quantity necessary for all tests required to determine that the active ingredient meets its established specifications.
Twice

YOUR COMPANY NAME

Name: _____ ID No.: _____ Issued by: _____

Designation: _____ Department: _____ Date: _____

17. All retention samples of active materials are to be retained for _____ after expiry of the last lot of the product containing the material.
One year

18. There must be a mechanism in place to assure _____ of retention samples.
Accountability

19. In case the _____ are used for investigation, documentation must be done to indicate reason for opening to keep the track of usage.
Retention samples

QCT-05.5

Assessment for Stability Analytical Methods and Requirements

YOUR COMPANY NAME

Name: _____ ID No.: _____ Issued by: _____

Designation: _____ Department: _____ Date: _____

1. The main purpose of performing stability studies is to collect _____ regarding the impact that environmental factors may have over the quality of drug substances and products.
   a. Samples
   b. Information
   c. Data
   d. Results

2. All regulatory agencies have emphasized on the significance of _____ which makes it a critical component of GMP.
   a. Accelerated stability study
   b. Stability study
   c. Humidity and temperature
   d. Data collection

3. Stability studies are considered important because _____.
   a. Help monitoring product quality
   b. Collection of data is possible
   c. Validation is not performed
   d. Customers demand for it

4. An SOP for stability study must be available at the site along with the presence of a _____.
   a. Stability master plan
   b. Stability protocol
   c. Stability chamber
   d. Stability laboratory

YOUR COMPANY NAME

Name: _____ ID No.: _____ Issued by: _____

Designation: _____ Department: _____ Date: _____

5. The stability protocol should address the testing schedule and plan in detail to comply with _____ written for each product.
   a. FDA requirements
   b. Company's policy
   c. NDA commitments
   d. Stability protocol

6. The stability procedures must define the sample size, test intervals and the number of lots to be tested based upon _____ to ensure valid estimates of stability.
   a. Statistical criteria
   b. Number of batches produced per year
   c. Types of dosage forms
   d. Batch size for each product

7. There must be a system through which the official SOPs related to stability studies are _____ in the laboratory.
   a. Released
   b. Controlled
   c. Written
   d. Retrieved

8. This should be a part of the system that the use of a _____ be prevented if the documented training has not taken place.
   a. New study
   b. New procedure
   c. New product
   d. New process

9. In order to implement a successful stability program, a procedure should be available to place at least one lot of each product/package on _____ each year.
   a. Annual review
   b. Stability
   c. Re-validation
   d. Testing

YOUR COMPANY NAME

Name: _____ ID No.: _____ Issued by: _____

Designation: _____ Department: _____ Date: _____

10. As per the stability procedure, after each NDA or ANDA approval, the first three lots must be _____.
    a. Validated
    b. Reviewed extensively
    c. Placed on stability
    d. Released for commercial use

11. The changes in formulation, drug substance, container closure, the manufacturing site or any type of reprocessing of material must be followed by the evaluation of _____.
    a. Batch documents
    b. Stability data
    c. Manufacturing equipment
    d. Manufacturing processes

12. In the solid dosage forms, the container _____ is also challenged by stressing the adhesive properties on higher then 70% RH and 30°C.
    a. Material
    b. Printing
    c. Sealant integrity
    d. Supplier

13. During the stability studies, the sample retrieval should be not more than one week prior to the due date and tested not more than _____ after the due date.
    a. One week
    b. Two weeks
    c. One month
    d. Two days

14. As per the stability protocol the testing is performed every three months over the first year, every six months over the second year and _____ thereafter.
    a. Every nine months
    b. Annually
    c. Every month
    d. 18 months

YOUR COMPANY NAME

Name: _____ ID No.: _____ Issued by: _____

Designation: _____ Department: _____ Date: _____

15. The time "zero" is defined as the first testing of the initial samples at the time of _____.
    a. Bulk testing
    b. Release
    c. First three months testing
    d. First year

16. To analyse the data, _____ should be calculated around the degradation curves based up on 95% of the label claim.
    a. Expiry date
    b. Confidence level
    c. Shelf life
    d. Potency of active ingredient

17. The stability study procedure should address the requirement that in case a 5% potency loss or OOS condition occurs at 40°C, 75%RH, then a study at _____ must be initiated and continued for 6 months.
    a. 30°C/45% RH
    b. 30°C/60% RH
    c. 3 months
    d. New samples

18. The issuance and controlling of stability _____ should be under an approved system.
    a. Samples
    b. Specifications
    c. Data
    d. Report

19. The testing requirements for appearance, friability, hardness, colour, odour, moisture, strength, and dissolution are for _____.
    a. Suspensions
    b. Capsules
    c. Tablets
    d. Ampoules

YOUR COMPANY NAME

Name: _____ ID No.: _____ Issued by: _____

Designation: _____ Department: _____ Date: _____

20. Reasonable intervals must be outlined in the stability procedure for sampling and testing of _____ for strength, appearance, colour, particulate matter, pH, sterility, and pyrogenicity.
    a. Large volume parenterals
    b. Small volume parenterals
    c. Lyophilized products
    d. Suppositories

21. All topical preparations in containers larger than 3.5 g will be sampled and tested at the surface, middle and bottom of the container to ensure _____ throughout the shelf life.
    a. Homogeneity
    b. Absence of topical pathogens
    c. Potency
    d. Smoothness

22. For _____, the specifications and testing requirements include delivered dose per actuation, number of doses, colour, clarity (solutions), particle size distribution (suspensions), loss of propellant, pressure, valve corrosion and spray pattern.
    a. Respiratory inhalers
    b. Syrup
    c. Injectables
    d. Capsules

23. As per stability study protocol the requirement to ensure that preservative content of applicable drug products is monitored at least at the beginning and end of the _____.
    a. Shelf life
    b. Stability study
    c. Manufacturing process
    d. Accelerated stability study

YOUR COMPANY NAME

Name: _____ ID No.: _____ Issued by: _____

Designation: _____ Department: _____ Date: _____

24. For a change control in stability study, same policy applies as for other controlled documents that prohibit any change except those _____ QA.
    a. Initiated by
    b. Authorized by
    c. Requested by
    d. Identified by

25. The proposal for a change in the quality standards for stability testing, its evaluation and implementation will be governed by a system, which will evaluate if a _____ of the method is deemed necessary after the change is implemented.
    a. Verification
    b. Transfer
    c. Re-validation
    d. Change

QCT-05.5.1

Answers to Quiz for Stability Analytical Methods and Requirements

YOUR COMPANY NAME

Name: _____ ID No.: _____ Issued by: _____

Designation: _____ Department: _____ Date: _____

1. The main purpose of performing stability studies is to collect _____ regarding the impact that environmental factors may have over the quality of drug substances and products.
   Information

2. All regulatory agencies have emphasized on the significance of _____ which makes it a critical component of GMP.
   Stability study

3. Stability studies are considered important because of _____.
   Help monitoring product quality

4. An SOP for stability study must be available at the site along with the presence of a _____.
   Stability protocol

5. The stability protocol should address the testing schedule and plan in detail to comply with _____ written for each product.
   NDA commitments

6. The stability procedures must define the sample size, test intervals and the number of lots to be tested based upon _____ to ensure valid estimates of stability.
   Statistical criteria

YOUR COMPANY NAME

Name: _____ ID No.: _____ Issued by: _____

Designation: _____ Department: _____ Date: _____

7. There must be a system through which the official SOPs related to stability studies are _____ in the laboratory.
Controlled

8. This should be a part of the system that the use of a _____ be prevented if the documented training has not taken place.
New procedure

9. In order to implement a successful stability program, a procedure should be available to place at least one lot of each product/package on _____ each year.
Stability

10. As per the stability procedure, after each NDA or ANDA approval, the first three lots must be _____.
Placed on stability

11. The changes in formulation, drug substance, container closure, the manufacturing site or any type of reprocessing of material must be followed by the evaluation of _____.
Stability data

12. In the solid dosage forms, the container _____ is also challenged by stressing the adhesive properties on higher then 70% RH and 30°C.
Sealant integrity

13. During the stability studies, the samples retrieval should be not more than one week prior to the due date and tested not more than _____ after the due date.
One month

14. As per the stability protocol the testing is performed every three months over the first year, every six months over the second year and _____ thereafter.
Annually

YOUR COMPANY NAME

Name: _____ ID No.: _____ Issued by: _____

Designation: _____ Department: _____ Date: _____

15. The time "zero" is defined as the first testing of the initial samples at the time of _____.
    Release

16. To analyse the data, _____ should be calculated around the degradation curves based upon 95% of the label claim.
    Confidence level

17. The stability study procedure should address the requirement that in case a 5% potency loss or OOS condition occurs at 40°C, 75%RH, then a study at _____ must be initiated and continued for 6 months.
    30°C/60% RH

18. The issuance and controlling of stability _____ should be under an approved system.
    Samples

19. The testing requirements for appearance, friability, hardness, colour, odour, moisture, strength, and dissolution are for _____.
    Tablets

20. Reasonable intervals must be outlined in the stability procedure for sampling and testing of _____ for strength, appearance, colour, particulate matter, pH, sterility, and pyrogenicity.
    Small-volume parenterals

21. All topical preparations in containers larger than 3.5 g will be sampled and tested at the surface, middle and bottom of the container to ensure _____ throughout the shelf life.
    Homogeneity

22. For _____, the specifications and testing requirements include delivered dose per actuation, number of doses, colour, clarity (solutions), particle size distribution (suspensions), loss of propellant, pressure, valve corrosion, and spray pattern.
    Respiratory inhalers

YOUR COMPANY NAME

Name: _____ ID No.: _____ Issued by: _____

Designation: _____ Department: _____ Date: _____

23. As per stability study protocol the requirement to ensure that preservative content of applicable drug products is monitored at least at the beginning and end of the _____.
    Stability study

24. For a change control in stability study, same policy applies as for other controlled documents that prohibit any change except those _____ QA.
    Authorized by

25. The proposal for a change in the quality standards for stability testing, its evaluation and implementation will be governed by a system, which will evaluate if a _____ of the method is deemed necessary after the change is implemented.
    Re-validation

QCT-05.6

Assessment for Microbiological Methods and Testing

YOUR COMPANY NAME

Name: _____ ID No.: _____ Issued by: _____

Designation: _____ Department: _____ Date: _____

1. Non-sterile products and raw materials of biological and botanical origin required to be tested for _____.
   a. Microbial limits
   b. Pathogens
   c. Sterility
   d. Physical appearance

2. All microbiological laboratories need to have a procedure to test the total number of microorganisms and to assess the absence of specific _____.
   a. Contaminants
   b. Bacterial species
   c. Impurities
   d. Ingredients

3. The microbiology department functions include monitoring/testing of the environment, compressed gases, water and _____.
   a. Media control
   b. Final release
   c. Aseptic filtration
   d. Maintenance of laminar flow

4. Where appropriate, microbiological testing methods must comply with _____.
   a. FDA requirements
   b. Finished products specifications
   c. NDA requirements
   d. Environmental requirements

YOUR COMPANY NAME

Name: _____ ID No.: _____ Issued by: _____

Designation: _____ Department: _____ Date: _____

5. The method used for demonstrating the ability of culture media to support the growth of microorganisms is called _____.
   a. Sterility test
   b. Process simulation test
   c. Growth promotion test
   d. Filter integrity test

6. There must be an SOP that prevents the use of media before it has been _____.
   a. Tested
   b. Approved
   c. Sterilized
   d. Sampled

7. The SOP must recommend performing the growth promotion testing with _____ normally found in the environment of a specific site or a manufacturing location within a site.
   a. Organisms
   b. People
   c. Material
   d. Equipment

8. An SOP always governs media preparation and also provides instructions on how to _____ media with a complete autoclave cycle definition.
   a. Use
   b. Purify
   c. Sterilize
   d. Release

9. Media have to be sterilized always in _____ autoclaves.
   a. Clean
   b. Qualified
   c. New
   d. Production's

YOUR COMPANY NAME

Name: _____ ID No.: _____ Issued by: _____

Designation: _____ Department: _____ Date: _____

10. Exhaust system, steam supply, pressure holds and initial jacket mapping study are some of the elements which must be included in _____ for autoclaves.
    a. Design qualification
    b. Installation qualification
    c. Calibration
    d. Daily maintenance

11. All thermometers and thermocouples used in the microbiology laboratory must be part of _____.
    a. Routine maintenance program
    b. Master calibration plan
    c. Inventory list
    d. Microbiology department

12. The Microbiology laboratory must have procedures describing the necessary _____ for microbiological and sterility testing.
    a. Sterilization techniques
    b. Aseptic techniques
    c. Analytical techniques
    d. Training

13. Design of door handles for use without touching palms is one of the important features for _____.
    a. Microbiology lab
    b. Gowning facility
    c. Chemical lab
    d. Shower area

14. The analyst's ability to properly gown should be evaluated by means of _____.
    a. Contact plate testing
    b. Visual testing
    c. Air particulate counter
    d. Media fill

YOUR COMPANY NAME

Name: _____ ID No.: _____ Issued by: _____

Designation: _____ Department: _____ Date: _____

15. Before performing a sterility test, analysts must ensure that the method being used is consistent with _____.
    a. NDA commitments
    b. Products specifications
    c. Validation protocol
    d. Growth promotion test result

16. Manipulated _____ should be used during each sterility test.
    a. Microorganisms
    b. Negative controls
    c. Reagents
    d. Methods

17. Type of organism and acceptance criteria for identification should be part of approved _____ prior to validation.
    a. Test method
    b. Specifications
    c. Protocol
    d. Report

18. The sterility test area must possess _____.
    a. Class 1000 environment
    b. Class 100 environment
    c. Wireless phone
    d. All required reagents

19. There should be an established _____ for environmental parameters in the sterility test area, with specified alert and action levels.
    a. Monitoring program
    b. Test method
    c. Operating procedure
    d. Policies and guidelines

20. The cleaning and disinfection procedures must be _____ for their effectiveness on specific surfaces and on specific organisms as well as their recovery studies from surfaces.
    a. Validated
    b. Checked
    c. Reviewed
    d. Guaranteed

QCT-05.6.1

Answers to Quiz for Microbiological Methods and Testing

YOUR COMPANY NAME

Name: _____ ID No.: _____ Issued by: _____

Designation: _____ Department: _____ Date: _____

1. Non-sterile products and raw materials of biological and botanical origin required to be tested for _____.
   Microbial limits

2. All microbiological laboratories need to have a procedure to test the total number of microorganisms and to assess the absence of specific _____.

   Bacterial species

3. The microbiology department functions include monitoring/testing of the environment, compressed gases, water, and _____.
   Media control

4. Where appropriate, microbiological testing methods must comply with _____.

   NDA requirements

5. The method used for demonstrating the ability of culture media to support the growth of microorganisms is called _____.
   Growth promotion test

6. There must be an SOP that prevents the use of media before it has been _____.

   Approved

YOUR COMPANY NAME

Name: _____ ID No.: _____ Issued by: _____

Designation: _____ Department: _____ Date: _____

7. The SOP must recommend performing the growth promotion testing with _____ normally found in the environment of a specific site or a manufacturing location within a site.
   Organisms

8. An SOP always governs media preparation and also provides instructions on how to _____ media with a complete autoclave cycle definition.
   Sterilize

9. Media have to be sterilized always in _____ autoclaves.
   Qualified

10. Exhaust system, steam supply, pressure holds and initial jacket mapping study are some of the elements, which must be included in _____ for autoclaves.
    Design qualification

11. All thermometers and thermocouples used in the microbiology laboratory must be part of _____.
    Master calibration plan

12. The microbiology laboratory must have procedures describing the necessary _____ for microbiological and sterility testing.
    Aseptic techniques

13. Design of door handles for use without touching palms is one of the important features for _____.
    Gowning facility

14. The analyst's ability to properly gown should be evaluated by means of _____.
    Contact plate testing

15. Before performing a sterility test, analysts must ensure that the method being used is consistent with _____.
    NDA commitments

YOUR COMPANY NAME

Name: _____ ID No.: _____ Issued by: _____

Designation: _____ Department: _____ Date: _____

16. Manipulated _____ should be used during each sterility test.
    Negative controls

17. Type of organism and acceptance criteria for identification should be part of approved _____ prior to validation.
    Protocol

18. The sterility test area must possess _____.
    Class 100 environments

19. There should be an established _____ for environmental parameters in the sterility test area, with specified alert and action levels.
    Monitoring program

20. The cleaning and disinfection procedures must be _____ for their effectiveness on specific surfaces and on specific organisms as well as their recovery studies from surfaces.
    Validated

QCT-05.7

Assessment for Laboratory Investigations

YOUR COMPANY NAME

Name: _____ ID No.: _____ Issued by: _____

Designation: _____ Department: _____ Date: _____

Fill in the blanks with appropriate answers from the multiple choices:

1. Laboratory investigations are _____ that is performed in the laboratory following an OOS or questionable result.
   a. GMP requirement
   b. Documented assessment
   c. Manager's responsibility
   d. Formality

2. OOS results can arise from cause, which can be divided into three categories: laboratory error, process-related error, and _____.
   a. Non-robust method
   b. Non-process-related error
   c. Analyst error
   d. Equipment failure

3. The objective of the procedure for OOS results investigations should be to determine if the OOS is _____.
   a. Unique
   b. Coincidence
   c. Valid
   d. Isolated incidence

4. According to the procedure, upon finding an OOS result, the analyst must inform the _____.
   a. Senior colleague
   b. Immediate supervisor
   c. Director quality assurance
   d. Production manager

YOUR COMPANY NAME

Name: _____ ID No.: _____ Issued by: _____

Designation: _____ Department: _____ Date: _____

5. Upon finding that the result is valid, the objective is to determine
   _____ and its impact.
   a. Who was the analyst
   b. The probable root cause
   c. The fate of the batch under question
   d. The probable disposition of the batch

6. It will be the responsibility of the immediate supervisor to assess the
   _____ and make a decision to inform the QC manager and
   production manager.
   a. Analyst's report
   b. Nature of problem
   c. Products history
   d. Manufacturing processes

7. The first stage of the procedure is laboratory investigation to determine
   if the OOS result is _____.
   a. Laboratory error
   b. Manufacturing error
   c. Equipment error
   d. False incident

8. Reviewing instruments calibration and maintenance records is a step of
   investigation that is conducted during the _____.
   a. Expanded investigation
   b. Laboratory investigation
   c. Maintenance department's investigation
   d. Analysts personal investigation

9. If the result of the initial laboratory investigation is inconclusive,
   _____.
   a. Batch should be immediately discarded
   b. A full-scale laboratory investigation is required
   c. Analyst should be re-trained
   d. Production operator should be re-trained

YOUR COMPANY NAME

Name: _____ ID No.: _____ Issued by: _____

Designation: _____ Department: _____ Date: _____

10. The initial retest must be performed by a second analyst _____
    using independently prepared solutions and a new instrument.
    a. Two times
    b. Three times
    c. Once
    d. On a second sample

11. The procedure should also address the involvement of _____ in
    the expanded investigation to determine the root cause for an OOS
    result.
    a. Quality assurance
    b. QC manager
    c. The first analyst
    d. Machine operator

12. A review of the information available about the material under test must
    be conducted as part of the _____.
    a. Initial investigation
    b. Expanded investigation
    c. Laboratory investigation
    d. Analyst's training

13. The OOS standard operating procedure must address _____ and
    consideration for corrective action to prevent recurrence.
    a. Re-issuance of new batch
    b. Rejection of batch
    c. Decision for re-working
    d. Preparation of fresh standards

14. In case the batch proves to be compliant as a result of retesting,
    _____.
    a. Specific directives must be present for disposition of batch
    b. Batch must still be rejected
    c. Batch should be re-worked
    d. Analysts should be re-trained not to report false incidence

YOUR COMPANY NAME

Name: _____ ID No.: _____ Issued by: _____

Designation: _____ Department: _____ Date: _____

15. As per the procedure, all the samples and reagents will be retained until the _____ has been completed.
    a. Next lot analysis
    b. Investigation
    c. Analysts training
    d. Analysis

16. The effectiveness of training on _____ must be measured by competency and performance objectives of the individuals.
    a. Analytical instruments
    b. Incidents report
    c. OOS investigations procedure
    d. Standards and reagents preparation

17. There must be a list of _____ for each training module that describes what the analyst is expected to learn upon completion of a training activity.
    a. Analytical instruments
    b. Expected results
    c. SOPs
    d. Analysts

18. The conclusions of OOS investigations and actions taken must be documented in a _____.
    a. Interim report
    b. Final report
    c. Standard operating procedure
    d. Training report

19. The SOP training documentation must be available in the _____ training file.
    a. Company's
    b. Employee's
    c. Instruments
    d. QA department's

YOUR COMPANY NAME

Name: _____ ID No.: _____ Issued by: _____

Designation: _____ Department: _____ Date: _____

20. The _____ must contain as a minimum the name and title of
    attendee, ID number, department, name of the instructor, date and time
    of training, duration of training session (hours and days) and training
    records, and so on.
    a. Training documentation
    b. Investigation report
    c. OOS procedure
    d. Employee's personal file

QCT-05.7.1

Answers to Quiz for Laboratory Investigations

YOUR COMPANY NAME

Name: _____ ID No.: _____ Issued by: _____

Designation: _____ Department: _____ Date: _____

1. Laboratory investigations are _____ that is performed in the laboratory following an OOS or questionable result.
   GMP requirement

2. OOS results can arise from cause, which can be divided into three categories: laboratory error, process-related error, and _____.
   Non-process-related error

3. The objective of the procedure for OOS results investigations should be to determine if the OOS result is _____.
   Valid

4. According to the procedure, up on finding an OOS result, the analyst must inform the _____.
   Immediate supervisor

5. Up on finding that the result is valid, the objective is to determine _____ and its impact.
   The probable root cause

6. It will be the responsibility of the immediate supervisor to assess the _____ and make a decision to inform the QC manager and production manager.
   Nature of problem

7. The first stage of the procedure is laboratory investigation to determine if the OOS result is _____.
   Laboratory error

YOUR COMPANY NAME

Name: _____ ID No.: _____ Issued by: _____

Designation: _____ Department: _____ Date: _____

8. Reviewing instruments calibration and maintenance records is a step of
   investigation that is conducted during the _____.
   Expanded investigation

9. If the result of the initial laboratory investigation is inconclusive,
   _____.
   A full-scale laboratory investigation is required

10. The initial retest must be performed by a second analyst _____
    using independently prepared solutions and a new instrument.
    Three times

11. The procedure should also address the involvement of _____ in
    the expanded investigation to determine the root cause for an OOS
    result.
    Quality assurance

12. A review of the information available about the material under test must
    be conducted as part of the _____.
    Expanded investigation

13. The OOS standard operating procedure must address _____ and
    consideration for corrective action to prevent recurrence.
    Rejection of batch

14. In case the batch proves to be compliant as a result of retesting,
    _____.
    Specific directives must be present for disposition of batch

15. As per the procedure, all the samples and reagents will be retained until
    the _____ has been completed.
    Investigation

16. The effectiveness of training on _____ must be measured by
    competency and performance objectives of the individuals.
    OOS investigations procedure

YOUR COMPANY NAME

Name: _____ ID No.: _____ Issued by: _____

Designation: _____ Department: _____ Date: _____

17. There must be a list of _____ for each training module that describes what the analyst is expected to learn upon completion of a training activity.
    Expected results

18. The conclusions of OOS investigations and actions taken must be documented in a _____.
    Final report

19. The SOP training documentation must be available in the _____ training file.
    Employees

20. The _____ must contain as a minimum the name title of attendee, ID number, department, name of the instructor, date and time of training, duration of training session (hours and days) and training records, and so on.
    Training documentation

QCT-05.8
Assessment for Calibration Programme

YOUR COMPANY NAME

Name: _____ ID No.: _____ Issued by: _____

Designation: _____ Department: _____ Date: _____

1. Calibration is a comparison between measurements of _____ and measurement made in as similar a way as possible with a second device.
   a. Instruments
   b. Known magnitude
   c. Performance
   d. Standard device

2. The calibration process begins with the _____ of the measuring instrument that needs to be calibrated.
   a. Design
   b. Quality
   c. Brand
   d. Model

3. In pharmaceutical QC laboratories, an instrument is considered calibrated as long as it returns values that are within predetermined specifications when compared against _____.
   a. Unknown quantities
   b. Known quantities
   c. Specified limits
   d. Non-calibrated instrument

4. QC laboratories should ensure that all analytical instruments are capable of _____.
   a. Testing as per STMs
   b. Producing valid and reproducible results
   c. Working automatically
   d. Producing results

YOUR COMPANY NAME

Name: _____ ID No.: _____ Issued by: _____

Designation: _____ Department: _____ Date: _____

5. The intent of the GMP calibration requirements is to assure adequate
   and continuous performance of measurement equipment with respect to
   _____ and _____, and so on.
   a. Accuracy; precision
   b. Compliance; conformance
   c. STMs; specifications
   d. Validation protocol; reports

6. _____ must be established to conduct calibration of all critical
   instruments in QC and microbiology laboratories.
   a. Expertise
   b. Standards
   c. Written procedures
   d. Justification

7. All instruments/equipment must be calibrated and re-qualified as per
   pre-determined intervals defined in the _____.
   a. Standard methods
   b. Calibration plan
   c. Laboratory plan
   d. Maintenance program

8. Maintenance department is responsible to initiate a _____,
   which should also include all instruments used in the QC laboratory.
   a. Master calibration plan
   b. Calibration procedure
   c. Instruments list
   d. Maintenance and preventive program

9. When a new instrument is included in QC lab, a request is initiated by
   the laboratory manager or supervisor for _____ to log in the new
   instrument in the calibration master plan.
   a. Purchase department
   b. Quality assurance department
   c. A senior analyst
   d. Maintenance department

YOUR COMPANY NAME

Name: _____ ID No.: _____ Issued by: _____

Designation: _____ Department: _____ Date: _____

10. As a minimum, the information such as system ID, description, equipment type and location, and so on, must be part of _____.
    a. Master calibration schedule
    b. Calibration procedure
    c. Instruments manual
    d. Quality control instruments list

11. Frequency, required equipment and standards, limits for accuracy and precision, preliminary examinations and operations, and calibration process description are as a minimum the information that must be part of _____.
    a. Calibration report
    b. Calibration procedure
    c. Qualification protocol
    d. Master instrument list

12. As per the calibration SOP, the calibration frequency for each instrument, provided by the _____, should be included in the calibration procedure of the particular instrument.
    a. Maintenance department
    b. Equipment manual
    c. Manufacturer
    d. Supplier

13. The manufacturer's frequency will be added to the Master Calibration Programme, which must be adhered to unless a _____ is deemed necessary.
    a. Re-validation
    b. Change
    c. Repair
    d. Training

14. If a change in equipment takes place, all the instruments associated with it will be _____ before reusing the system.
    a. Calibrated
    b. Changed
    c. Repaired
    d. Renewed

YOUR COMPANY NAME

Name: _____ ID No.: _____ Issued by: _____

Designation: _____ Department: _____ Date: _____

15. Any instrument, that is removable for _____ will be removed by the QC department's personnel and handed over to maintenance department.
    a. Maintenance
    b. Change of location
    c. Calibration
    d. Cleaning

16. In case an equipment/system has passed the due date for calibration, a "Do not use/Out of calibration" sticker must be immediately placed on it by _____.
    a. Laboratory supervisor or manager
    b. Maintenance manager
    c. Laboratory analyst
    d. QA inspector

17. All the calibration record will be kept in the corresponding binder, marked for the specific piece of equipment/instrument with _____ department.
    a. Maintenance
    b. Quality control
    c. Quality assurance
    d. Human resource

18. Clear instruction must be added to the calibration SOP as to how _____ will assess the impact on products quality if an out of calibration instrument is accidently used in the analysis.
    a. Quality control
    b. Maintenance
    c. QC manager
    d. Quality assurance

19. As per calibration SOP, if a non-scheduled calibration comes up the _____ must inform the maintenance department, in written, and request to perform calibration.
    a. Maintenance manager
    b. Equipment owner
    c. Calibration co-ordinator
    d. QC analyst

YOUR COMPANY NAME

Name: _____ ID No.: _____ Issued by: _____

Designation: _____ Department: _____ Date: _____

20. The calibration co-ordinator will follow up and make sure that the calibration is performed accurately, calibration record is completed and _____ is updated accordingly.
    a. Calibration master plan
    b. Calibration SOP
    c. Instrument logbook
    d. Training file

QCT-05.8.1

Answers to Quiz for Calibration Programme

YOUR COMPANY NAME

Name: _____ ID No.: _____ Issued by: _____

Designation: _____ Department: _____ Date: _____

1. Calibration is a comparison between measurements of _____ and measurement made in as similar a way as possible with a second device.
   Known magnitude

2. The calibration process begins with the _____ of the measuring instrument that needs to be calibrated.
   Design

3. In pharmaceutical QC laboratories, an instrument is considered calibrated as long as it returns values that are within predetermined specifications when compared against _____.
   Known quantities

4. QC laboratories should ensure that all analytical instruments are capable of _____.
   Producing valid and reproducible results

5. The intent of the GMP calibration requirements is to assure adequate and continuous performance of measurement equipment with respect to _____ and _____, and so on.
   Accuracy; Precision

6. _____ must be established to conduct calibration of all critical instruments in QC and microbiology laboratories.
   Written procedures

YOUR COMPANY NAME

Name: _____ ID No.: _____ Issued by: _____

Designation: _____ Department: _____ Date: _____

7. All instruments/equipment must be calibrated and re-qualified as per predetermined intervals defined in the _____.
   Calibration plan

8. Maintenance department is responsible to initiate a _____, which should also include all instruments used in the QC laboratory.
   Master calibration plan

9. When a new instrument is included in QC lab, a request is initiated by the laboratory manager or supervisor for _____ to log in the new instrument in the calibration master plan.
   Maintenance department

10. As a minimum, the information such as system ID, description, equipment type and location, and so on, must be part of _____.
    Master calibration schedule

11. Frequency, required equipment and standards, limits for accuracy and precision, preliminary examinations and operations, and calibration process description are as a minimum the information that must be part of _____.

    Calibration procedure

12. As per the calibration SOP, the calibration frequency for each instrument, provided by the _____, should be included in the calibration procedure of the particular instrument.
    Manufacturer

13. The manufacturer's frequency will be added to the master calibration programme, which must be adhered to unless a _____ is deemed necessary.
    Change

14. If a change in equipment takes place, all the instruments associated with it will be _____ before re-using the system.
    Calibrated

YOUR COMPANY NAME

Name: _____ ID No.: _____ Issued by: _____

Designation: _____ Department: _____ Date: _____

15. Any instrument that is removable for _____ will be removed by the QC department's personnel and handed over to maintenance department.
    Calibration

16. In case an equipment/system has passed due date for calibration, a "Do not use/Out of calibration" sticker must be immediately placed on it by _____.
    Laboratory supervisor or manager

17. All the calibration record will be kept in the corresponding binder, marked for the specific piece of equipment/instrument with _____ department.
    Quality control

18. Clear instruction must be added to the calibration SOP as to how _____ will assess the impact on products quality if an out-of-calibration instrument is accidentally used in the analysis.
    Quality assurance

19. As per calibration SOP, if a non-scheduled calibration comes up, the _____ must inform the maintenance department, in written, and request to perform calibration.
    Equipment owner

20. The calibration co-ordinator will follow up and make sure that the calibration is performed accurately, calibration record is completed and _____ is updated accordingly.
    Calibration master plan

QCT-05.9

Assessment for Laboratory Facility

YOUR COMPANY NAME

Name: _____ ID No.: _____ Issued by: _____

Designation: _____ Department: _____ Date: _____

1. Size, construction, and location, _____, housekeeping and personnel practices to facilitate cleaning, maintenance and proper operations are necessary for the area used for conducting the laboratory testing.
   a. Environmental conditions
   b. Cooling
   c. Heating
   d. Coziness

2. Adequate space should be available for the orderly placement of _____ to avoid congestion.
   a. Furniture
   b. Bottles of reagents
   c. Analytical instrument
   d. Laboratory logbooks

3. The laboratory must have a _____ area for storage of samples, which are to be tested, or are under testing.
   a. Big
   b. Separate
   c. Air-conditioned
   d. Non-dedicated

4. QC laboratory must have an instrument room where _____ instrument may be located.
   a. Only new
   b. Uncalibrated
   c. HPLC and GC
   d. Out of order

YOUR COMPANY NAME

Name: _____ ID No.: _____ Issued by: _____

Designation: _____ Department: _____ Date: _____

5. The design of the _____ must provide an adequate degree of
separation of the different activities to assure proper conduct of testing.
   a. Sampling room
   b. Test facility
   c. Instruments room
   d. Microbiology lab

6. Sufficient space in the microbiology laboratory will be required to install
_____ number of laminar flow hoods.
   a. Fewer
   b. Adequate
   c. Greater
   d. Minimum

7. Adequate _____ should be provided in all areas of laboratory to
facilitate proper functioning of the lab.
   a. Lighting
   b. Music
   c. Number of people
   d. Reagents

8. Equipment for the control and monitoring of air pressure, microorganisms, dust, humidity and temperature should also be provided especially
for the _____.
   a. Manager's office
   b. Sample storage area
   c. Microbiological laboratory
   d. Archive room

9. _____ water should be supplied under continuous positive pressure in a plumbing system free from defects.
   a. Ultra purified
   b. City
   c. Potable
   d. WFI

YOUR COMPANY NAME

Name: _____ ID No.: _____ Issued by: _____

Designation: _____ Department: _____ Date: _____

10. The laboratory area must have a safe storage for _____ materials.
    a. Expensive
    b. Hazardous
    c. USP
    d. In-process

11. A written procedure must be established to address handling of _____ after testing.
    a. Mobile phase
    b. Remaining samples
    c. Reference standards
    d. Volumetric solution

12. As per the standard operating procedure, all remaining samples after complete analyses will be treated as _____.
    a. Reference samples
    b. Pharmaceutical waste
    c. Stock samples
    d. Free to take home

13. Dry products and remaining packaging material will be put in plastic trash bags or carton boxes labelled clearly _____.
    a. "Pharmaceutical waste"
    b. "Do not waste"
    c. "Hazardous material"
    d. "Do not touch"

14. The pharmaceutical waste is transferred to the pharmaceutical waste area from where it is picked up by _____ people to dump.
    a. Common
    b. Production
    c. Municipality
    d. Quality assurance

YOUR COMPANY NAME

Name: _____ ID No.: _____ Issued by: _____

Designation: _____ Department: _____ Date: _____

15. Archive room for the storage and retrieval of raw data, reports, and samples should be available either in the same laboratory or in a _____.
    a. Satellite facility
    b. Other laboratory
    c. Far-flung area
    d. Restricted area

16. Samples of raw and packaging materials and finished products should be arranged in _____ according to the batch number for easy tracking.
    a. A shelf
    b. Serial numbers
    c. A separate room
    d. The manager's office

17. The temperature and humidity readings in the reference samples room must be monitored on _____ basis and recorded in a logbook.
    a. Monthly
    b. Weekly
    c. Daily
    d. Hourly

18. There should be controlled access to retention and stability samples room and a _____ should be maintained to control the entry of personnel in these areas.
    a. Close circuit camera
    b. Logbook
    c. Code word
    d. Lock and key

19. A written procedure must be established for the proper storage of _____ so as to minimize loss of viability.
    a. Reference standards
    b. Growth media
    c. Bacterial strains
    d. Reagents

YOUR COMPANY NAME

Name: _____ ID No.: _____ Issued by: _____

Designation: _____ Department: _____ Date: _____

20. The microbiological areas must be cleaned by 5% sodium hypochlorite (1:8 dilution) before and after finishing each _____ in the lab.
    a. Sterility test
    b. Microbiological growth test
    c. Shift
    d. Autoclaving

21. Solution of 3% _____ should be used to disinfect the working surfaces of microbiology lab at least once a week.
    a. H_2O_2
    b. NaOH
    c. Isopropyl alcohol
    d. Ethanol

22. For cleaning sterility testing room, only _____ solutions and disinfectants should be used.
    a. Diluted
    b. Concentrated
    c. Freshly prepared
    d. Valid

23. Incubators and refrigerators in the microbiology lab must be cleaned as per procedure once a month, whereas in the chemical lab cleaning of these equipments should be done once in _____.
    a. Three months
    b. Three weeks
    c. A year
    d. Two months

24. Laboratory glassware should be washed when required, with _____ cleansing mixture (ref. USP 30).
    a. Sulphuric acid
    b. Nitric acid
    c. Chromic acid
    d. Sodium hydroxide

YOUR COMPANY NAME

Name: _____ ID No.: _____ Issued by: _____

Designation: _____ Department: _____ Date: _____

25. To ensure proper functioning of the safety shower, periodic check must
    be done, preferably every _____.
    a. Week
    b. Day
    c. Month
    d. Hour

QCT-05.9.1

Answers to Quiz for Laboratory Facility

YOUR COMPANY NAME

Name: _____ ID No.: _____ Issued by: _____

Designation: _____ Department: _____ Date: _____

1. Size, construction and location, _____, housekeeping and personnel practices to facilitate cleaning, maintenance and proper operations are necessary for the area used for conducting the laboratory testing.
   Environmental conditions

2. Adequate space should be available for the orderly placement of _____ to avoid congestion.
   Analytical instrument

3. The laboratory must have a _____ area for storage of samples, which are to be tested, or are under testing.
   Separate

4. QC laboratory must have an instrument room where _____ instrument may be located.
   HPLC and GC

5. The design of the _____ must provide an adequate degree of separation of the different activities to assure proper conduct of testing.
   Test facility

6. Sufficient space in the microbiology laboratory will be required to install _____ number of laminar flow hoods.
   Adequate

7. Adequate _____ should be provided in all areas of laboratory to facilitate proper functioning of the lab.
   Lighting

YOUR COMPANY NAME

Name: _____ ID No.: _____ Issued by: _____

Designation: _____ Department: _____ Date: _____

8. Equipment for the control and monitoring of air pressure, microorganisms, dust, humidity and temperature should also be provided especially for the _____.
   Microbiological laboratory

9. _____ water should be supplied under continuous positive pressure in a plumbing system free from defects.
   Potable

10. The laboratory area must have a safe storage for _____ materials.
    Hazardous

11. A written procedure must be established to address handling of _____ after testing.
    Remaining samples

12. As per the standard operating procedure, all remaining samples after complete analyses will be treated as _____.
    Pharmaceutical waste

13. Dry products and remaining packaging material will be put in plastic trash bags or carton boxes labelled clearly _____.
    "Pharmaceutical waste"

14. The pharmaceutical waste is transferred to the pharmaceutical waste area from where it is picked up by _____ people to dump.
    Municipality

15. Archive room for the storage and retrieval of raw data, reports, and samples should be available either in the same laboratory or in a _____.
    Satellite facility

16. Samples of raw and packaging materials and finished products should be arranged in _____ according to the batch number for easy tracking.
    Serial numbers

YOUR COMPANY NAME

Name: _____ ID No.: _____ Issued by: _____

Designation: _____ Department: _____ Date: _____

17. The temperature and humidity readings in the reference samples room must be monitored on _____ basis and recorded in a logbook.
    Daily

18. There should be controlled access to retention and stability samples room and a _____ should be maintained to control the entry of personnel in these areas.
    Logbook

19. The written procedure must be established for the proper storage of _____ so as to minimize loss of viability.
    Bacterial strains

20. The microbiological areas must be cleaned by 5% sodium hypochlorite (1:8 dilution) before and after finishing each _____ in the lab.
    Shift

21. Solution of 3% _____ should be used to disinfect the working surfaces of the microbiology lab at least once a week.
    H_2O_2

22. For cleaning sterility testing room, only _____ solutions and disinfectants should be used.
    Freshly prepared

23. Incubators and refrigerators in the microbiology lab must be cleaned as per the procedure once a month, whereas in the chemical lab cleaning of these equipments should be done once in _____.
    Three months

24. Laboratory glassware should be washed when required, with _____ cleansing mixture (ref. USP 30).
    Chromic acid

25. To ensure proper functioning of the safety shower, periodic check must be done, preferably every _____.
    Week

QCT-05.10

Assessment for Annual Reviews

YOUR COMPANY NAME

Name: _____ ID No.: _____ Issued by: _____

Designation: _____ Department: _____ Date: _____

1. Annual product reviews process is established to determine the need for _____ in drug products specifications, manufacturing or control procedures.
   a. Validation
   b. Change
   c. Analysis
   d. Deviations

2. The site must develop and adhere to the _____ for annual product reviews detailing all required information and evaluation elements.
   a. Standard operating procedure
   b. Policy
   c. Guidelines
   d. Techniques

3. As per the SOP, QA and QC, product development and _____ are usually involved in the provision and compilation of data.
   a. Computer department
   b. Maintenance department
   c. Planning department
   d. Purchase department

4. After 60 days of the anniversary of _____ the annual review of the corresponding product will have to be completed.
   a. Product
   b. NDA/ANDA
   c. Expiry date
   d. First lot

YOUR COMPANY NAME

Name: _____ ID No.: _____ Issued by: _____

Designation: _____ Department: _____ Date: _____

5. Critical data for both _____ and finished product should be collected, accurately transcribed, analysed and compared to the corresponding specifications.
   a. Active ingredient
   b. Excipients
   c. Manufacturing intermediates
   d. Bulk

6. Annual reviews should also include an executive summary of the product manufacturing experience during the _____.
   a. Manufacturing of first lot
   b. Review period
   c. Manufacturing of most recent lot
   d. Shelf life

7. As per procedure, each _____, a collective report based on quantitative and qualitative results of all test will be published for each product.
   a. Subsequent year
   b. Quarter
   c. Month
   d. Two years

8. The review conclusion must not be delayed by more than the_____ of next year.
   a. First month
   b. First quarter
   c. Second quarter
   d. Two weeks

9. The review input and comments along with any _____ should be included on the form and attach with the finished product reports.
   a. Recommendations
   b. Corrective action
   c. Change in process
   d. Change in specification

YOUR COMPANY NAME

Name: _____ ID No.: _____ Issued by: _____

Designation: _____ Department: _____ Date: _____

10. It is the responsibility of _____ to forward final reports requiring corrective actions to respective departments for the implementation.
    a. QA manager
    b. QC manager
    c. Validation co-ordinator
    d. Change control co-ordinator

11. The appropriate management from manufacturing, technical services/operations, QC and _____ departments must review these annual reviews.
    a. Planning
    b. Regulatory
    c. Validation
    d. Maintenance

12. All records will be retained by _____ department.
    a. Quality assurance
    b. Quality control
    c. Production
    d. Validation

13. In order to assure _____, a second check should always be performed on data transcribed as part of annual review.
    a. Quality
    b. Reliability
    c. Good review
    d. Better report

14. Ongoing data capture, trending and _____ analysis must be carried on continued basis.
    a. Technical
    b. Chemical
    c. Physical
    d. Statistical

YOUR COMPANY NAME

Name: _____ ID No.: _____ Issued by: _____

Designation: _____ Department: _____ Date: _____

15. There must be clear guidelines in the written procedure for further
    _____ if anomalies are found in any of the data reviewed or in
    the resulting analysis.
    a. Reviews
    b. Investigations
    c. Analysis
    d. Discussions

QCT-05.10.1

Answers to Quiz for Annual Reviews

Name: _____ ID No.: _____ Issued by: _____

Designation: _____ Department: _____ Date: _____

1. Annual product review process is established to determine the need for _____ in drug products specifications, manufacturing or control procedures.
   Change

2. The site must develop and adhere to the _____ for annual product reviews detailing all required information and evaluation elements.
   Standard operating procedure

3. As per the SOP, QA, QC, product development and _____ are usually involved in the provision and compilation of data.
   Computer department

4. After 60 days of the anniversary of _____ the annual review of the corresponding product will have to be completed.
   NDA/ANDA

5. Critical data for both _____ and finished product should be collected, accurately transcribed, analysed and compared to the corresponding specifications.
   Manufacturing intermediates

6. Annual reviews should also include an executive summary of the product manufacturing experience during the _____.
   Review period

YOUR COMPANY NAME

Name: _____ ID No.: _____ Issued by: _____

Designation: _____ Department: _____ Date: _____

7. As per procedure, each _____, a collective report based on quantitative and qualitative results of all test will be published for each product.
   Subsequent year

8. The review conclusion must not be delayed by more than the _____ of next year.
   First month

9. The review input and comments along with any _____ should be included on the form and attach with the finished product reports.
   Corrective action

10. It is the responsibility of _____ to forward final reports requiring corrective actions to respective departments for the implementation.
    QA manager

11. The appropriate management from manufacturing, technical services/operations, QC and _____ departments must review these annual reviews.
    Validation

12. All records will be retained by _____ department.
    Quality assurance

13. In order to assure _____, a second check should always be performed on data transcribed as part of annual review.
    Reliability

14. Ongoing data capture, trending and _____ analysis must be carried on continued basis.
    Statistical

15. There must be clear guidelines in the written procedure for further _____ if anomalies are found in any of the data reviewed or in the resulting analysis.
    Investigations

QCT-05.11

Assessment for Third-Party Testing

YOUR COMPANY NAME

Name: _____ ID No.: _____ Issued by: _____

Designation: _____ Department: _____ Date: _____

1. Health regulatory agencies in the United States _____ hundreds of products each year to prevent injury to customers.
   a. Manufacture
   b. Market
   c. Develop
   d. Recall

2. Companies involved in a product recall have to face a series of impacts and need to take a number of _____.
   a. Corrective actions
   b. Tough decisions
   c. People for employment
   d. Development projects

3. As a corrective action to product recall, companies may have to change product design and packaging, withdraw products from the distribution channels, and offer _____ to the affected.
   a. Medical assistance
   b. Replacements
   c. Help
   d. Counselling

4. The most preferable time for third-party testing is while a product is in the _____ stage.
   a. Design
   b. Manufacturing
   c. Packaging stage
   d. Development

YOUR COMPANY NAME

Name: _____ ID No.: _____ Issued by: _____

Designation: _____ Department: _____ Date: _____

5. The third-party testing provides an independent check and balance to ensure that the outsourcer is delivering a product that will not surprise and frustrate its _____ at a later time.
   a. Developers
   b. Business partners
   c. Advisors
   d. Users

6. One of the reasons for having a third-party testing is that many laboratories do not have the _____ required to conduct a certain type of analysis.
   a. Money
   b. Expertize
   c. Desire
   d. Space

7. A service level _____ must exist between the third-party lab and the client.
   a. Agreement
   b. Contacts
   c. Partnership
   d. Friendship

8. One of the major benefits of third-party testing to the pharmaceutical industries could be reducing the _____ of client lab.
   a. Workload
   b. Risk of financial loss
   c. Waste of reagents and solutions
   d. Use of analytical instruments

9. The third-party testing also saves rework time by reducing _____ in the first place.
   a. People
   b. Errors
   c. Machines
   d. Standards

YOUR COMPANY NAME

Name: _____ ID No.: _____ Issued by: _____

Designation: _____ Department: _____ Date: _____

10. The laboratory must establish a system, which clearly defines the
    _____ of both parties.
    a. Qualification
    b. Expertise
    c. Responsibilities
    d. Identification

11. The customer lab must conduct _____ of the third-party labora-
    tories through an established mechanism.
    a. Training
    b. Periodic audit
    c. Gap analysis
    d. Evaluation

12. The customer laboratory should verify _____ taken as a result
    of inspections done by a health regulatory body or GMP authority.
    a. Achievements
    b. Qualifications
    c. Corrective measures
    d. Suggestions

13. If the customer's lab test methods are intended for testing, then the sys-
    tem must be in place to first carry out _____ of those quality test
    methods.
    a. Experiment
    b. Methods transfer
    c. Instruments qualification
    d. Evaluation

14. For third-party testing, a system must be formulated to delineate
    _____ from the third party to the customer's lab.
    a. Data reporting
    b. Sample transportation
    c. Results review
    d. Reagents

YOUR COMPANY NAME

Name: _____ ID No.: _____ Issued by: _____

Designation: _____ Department: _____ Date: _____

15. The written procedure should also define the responsibilities for data review as well as acceptance and rejection of the _____ at the third-party lab.
    a. Data
    b. Results
    c. Samples
    d. Lots

QCT-05.11.1

Answers to Quiz for Third-Party Testing

YOUR COMPANY NAME

Name: _____ ID No.: _____ Issued by: _____

Designation: _____ Department: _____ Date: _____

1. Health regulatory agencies in the United States _____ hundreds of products each year to prevent injury to customers.
   Recall

2. Companies involved in a product recall have to face a series of impacts and need to take a number of _____.
   Corrective actions

3. As a corrective action to product recall, companies may have to change product design and packaging, withdraw products from the distribution channels, and offer _____ to the affected.
   Replacements

4. The most preferable time for third-party testing is while a product is in the _____ stage.
   Design

5. The third-party testing provides an independent check and balance to ensure that the outsourcer is delivering a product that will not surprise and frustrate its _____ at a later time.
   Users

6. One of the reasons for having a third-party testing is that many laboratories do not have the _____ required to conduct a certain type of analysis.
   Expertise

YOUR COMPANY NAME

Name: _____ ID No.: _____ Issued by: _____

Designation: _____ Department: _____ Date: _____

7. A service level _____ must exist between the third-party lab and the client.
   Agreement

8. One of the major benefits of third-party testing to the pharmaceutical industries could be reducing the _____ of client lab.
   Workload

9. The third-party testing also saves rework time by reducing _____ in the first place.
   Errors

10. The laboratory must establish a system, which clearly defines the _____ of both parties.
    Responsibilities

11. The customer lab must conduct _____ of the third-party laboratories through an established mechanism.
    Periodic audit

12. The customer laboratory should verify _____ taken as a result of inspections done by a health regulatory body or GMP authority.
    Corrective measures

13. If the customer's lab test methods are intended for testing, then system must be in place to first carry out _____ of those quality test methods.
    Methods transfer

14. For third-party testing, a system must be formulated to delineate _____ from the third-party to the customer's lab.
    Data reporting

15. The written procedure should also define the responsibilities for data review as well as acceptance and rejection of the _____ at the third-party lab.
    Data

QCT-05.12

Assessment for Good Documentation Practices

YOUR COMPANY NAME

Name: _____ ID No.: _____ Issued by: _____

Designation: _____ Department: _____ Date: _____

1. Documentation is a system, which manages and controls all _____ during various activities performed in a pharmaceutical organization.
   a. Activities
   b. Processes
   c. Documents
   d. Personnel

2. The purpose of _____ is to clearly document the actions that took place in the development, manufacture, testing and releasing for commercial use of a drug, biologics, vaccine, medical device, and so on.
   a. Good documentation practice
   b. Good manufacturing practice
   c. Good laboratory practice
   d. Standard operating procedures

3. A controlled record is considered a _____ document, hence the data need to be clearly documented for legal and preservation purposes.
   a. Unofficial
   b. Official
   c. Legal
   d. Personal

4. _____ is required to assure the safety, identity, strength, purity and quality of the drug product.
   a. Validation
   b. Quality control
   c. Documentation
   d. Training

YOUR COMPANY NAME

Name: _____ ID No.: _____ Issued by: _____

Designation: _____ Department: _____ Date: _____

5. The QC laboratory must have an SOP for the management and control of laboratory documentation related to _____
   a. Analytical functions
   b. Batch audit
   c. Instrument calibration
   d. Instrument qualification

6. The _____ at the site must outline the requirements for generation, review, approval and control of documents defining the receiving of samples, assigning work to analysts, testing and releasing of products.
   a. Guidelines
   b. Standard test methods
   c. Policies and procedures
   d. Employee's job description

7. Documentation control requirements must include a system for assigning and controlling _____ to SOPs and STMs.
   a. Names
   b. Titles
   c. Effective dates
   d. Issuance date

8. The procedure for distribution and control of _____ within the QC lab must be defined in the SOP.
   a. Standards
   b. Documents
   c. SOPs
   d. Data

9. Procedure also needs to emphasize that all records are secured, available and easily _____ throughout the retention period.
   a. Traceable
   b. Retrievable
   c. Protected
   d. Copied

YOUR COMPANY NAME

Name: _____ ID No.: _____ Issued by: _____

Designation: _____ Department: _____ Date: _____

10. The data must be entered directly in the _____ and not on a scrap paper for the interim period.
    a. Controlled record
    b. Note book
    c. Official register
    d. Manager's diary

11. Documents dates should be in _____ format as specified in the SOP
    a. International
    b. Standardized
    c. Basic
    d. English

12. Each page in the controlled notebook should be numbered _____.
    a. Alphabetically
    b. Chronologically
    c. Systematically
    d. Automatically

13. _____ all printouts related to analysis with initials and date.
    a. Keep in the safe
    b. Adhere to the notebook
    c. Store in the archive room
    d. Keep in the notebook

14. _____ use pencils or markers to record data in the notebook.
    a. Always
    b. Do not
    c. Sometimes
    d. Chemists always

15. All blank fields must be stricken out or put _____ with the analyst's initials and date.
    a. Not in use
    b. Not applicable
    c. Incorrect entry
    d. Blank

QCT-05.12.1

Answers to Quiz for Good Documentation Practices

YOUR COMPANY NAME

Name: _____ ID No.: _____ Issued by: _____

Designation: _____ Department: _____ Date: _____

1. Documentation is a system which manages and controls all _____ during various activities performed in a pharmaceutical organization.
   Documents

2. The purpose of _____ is to clearly document the actions took place in the development, manufacture, testing and releasing for commercial use of a drug, biologics, vaccine, medical device, and so on.
   Good documentation practice

3. A controlled record is considered a _____ document, so the data need to be clearly documented for legal and preservation purposes.
   Legal

4. _____ is required to assure the safety, identity, strength, purity and quality of the drug product.
   Documentation

5. The QC laboratory must have an SOP for the management and control of laboratory documentation related to _____.
   Analytical functions

6. The _____ at the site must outline the requirements for generation, review, approval and control of documents defining the receiving of samples, assigning work to analysts, testing and releasing of products.
   Policies and procedures

7. Documentation control requirements must include a system for assigning and controlling _____ to SOPs and STMs.
   Effective dates

YOUR COMPANY NAME

Name: _____ ID No.: _____ Issued by: _____

Designation: _____ Department: _____ Date: _____

8. The procedure for distribution and control of _____ within the QC lab must be defined in the SOP.
Documents

9. Procedure also needs to emphasize that all records are secured, available and easily _____ throughout the retention period.
Retrievable

10. The data must be entered directly in the _____ and not on a scrap paper for the interim period.
Controlled record

11. Document dates should be in _____ format as specified in the SOP.
Standardized

12. Each page in the controlled notebook should be numbered _____.
Chronologically

13. _____ for all printouts related to analysis with initials and date.
Adhere to the notebook

14. _____ use pencils or markers to record data in the notebook.
Do not

15. All blank fields must be stricken out or put _____ with the analyst's initials and date.
Not applicable

QCT-05.13

Assessment for Change Control

YOUR COMPANY NAME

Name: _____ ID No.: _____ Issued by: _____

Designation: _____ Department: _____ Date: _____

1. Change control is a _____ of reviewing and analysing the effect of a change and to ensure that system retains its validated status.
   a. Process
   b. Monitoring system
   c. License
   d. Sign

2. Change control is an important tool, which controls the change by _____ ownership of proposed change by qualified representative of appropriate discipline.
   a. Giving away
   b. Identifying
   c. Documenting
   d. Approving

3. _____ may be needed for a variety of reasons including new or improved functions and updating the technical documents as per current compendial references, and so on.
   a. Training
   b. Changes
   c. Documentation
   d. Procedure

4. According to the procedure, actions are taken if a _____ is proposed to existing analytical equipment or standard test method.
   a. Training
   b. New number
   c. Change
   d. New process

YOUR COMPANY NAME

Name: _____ ID No.: _____ Issued by: _____

Designation: _____ Department: _____ Date: _____

5. If a change is proposed to existing process that may affect product quality or _____ of the process, change control must be initiated.
   a. Authenticity
   b. Reproducibility
   c. Speed
   d. Total expenses

6. The purpose of change control process is to ensure the appropriate level of review, impact analysis, and approval _____ making any change in the approved systems.
   a. After
   b. During
   c. Before
   d. Without

7. Unplanned changes are actually deviations and should be addressed using _____ procedures.
   a. Deviation handling
   b. Incidents handling
   c. Change control
   d. Validation

8. Planned changes are intentional and _____ and can be permanent or temporary.
   a. Post approved
   b. Pre-approved
   c. Reviewed
   d. Well-thought of

9. Each document changed bears a revision number and a reason for revision, whereas the final document is reviewed and approved by _____ unit.
   a. Quality control
   b. Quality assurance
   c. Validation
   d. Production

YOUR COMPANY NAME

Name: _____ ID No.: _____ Issued by: _____

Designation: _____ Department: _____ Date: _____

10. STMs, raw material, finished product and packaging material specifications and analytical instruments are some examples of categories, which are _____ by the change control SOP.
    a. Governed
    b. Exempted
    c. Excluded
    d. Not governed

11. _____ of the lab can initiate the change request form unless otherwise instructed.
    a. Only manager
    b. Only supervisor
    c. Any person
    d. Senior-most analyst

12. The _____ must classify the change as minor, major and/or critical.
    a. Quality assurance
    b. Quality control
    c. Change initiating departmental head
    d. Change initiator

13. The change request form will be forwarded to the documentation control department for assigning _____.
    a. Responsible person
    b. Revision number
    c. Sequential number
    d. Reasons for change

14. The procedure must also outline the need of sending the change control form to _____ for their review and impact analysis.
    a. Quality assurance
    b. QA managers
    c. Other departments
    d. The initiator

YOUR COMPANY NAME

Name: _____ ID No.: _____ Issued by: _____

Designation: _____ Department: _____ Date: _____

15. The planned close out date will be placed on the _____ by initiator in consultation with all department effected by change.
    a. Department's notice board
    b. Original change control form
    c. Quality assurance monthly report
    d. Official memo

QCT-05.13.1

Answers to Quiz for Change Control

YOUR COMPANY NAME

Name: _____ ID No.: _____ Issued by: _____

Designation: _____ Department: _____ Date: _____

1. Change control is a _____ of reviewing and analysing the effect of a change and to ensure that system retains its validated status.
   Monitoring system

2. Change control is an important tool which controls the change by _____ ownership of proposed change by qualified representative of appropriate discipline.
   Identifying

3. _____ may be needed for a variety of reasons including new or improved functions and updating the technical documents as per current compendial references, and so on.
   Changes

4. According to the procedure, actions are taken if a _____ is proposed to existing analytical equipment or standard test method.
   Change

5. If a change is proposed to existing process that may affect product quality or _____ of the process, change control must be initiated.
   Reproducibility

6. The purpose of change control process is to ensure the appropriate level of review, impact analysis and approval _____ making any change in the approved systems.
   Before

YOUR COMPANY NAME

Name: _____ ID No.: _____ Issued by: _____

Designation: _____ Department: _____ Date: _____

7. Unplanned changes are actually deviations and should be addressed using _____ procedures.
   Deviation handling

8. Planned changes are intentional and _____ and can be permanent or temporary.
   Pre-approved

9. Each document changed bears a revision number and a reason for revision, whereas the final document is reviewed and approved by _____ unit.
   Quality assurance

10. STMs, raw material, finished product and packaging material specifications and analytical instruments are some examples of categories, which are _____ by the change control SOP.
    Governed

11. _____ of the lab can initiate the change request form unless otherwise instructed.
    Any person

12. The _____ must classify the change as minor, major and/or critical.
    Change initiating departmental head

13. The change request form will be forwarded to the documentation control department for assigning _____.
    Sequential number

14. The procedure must also outline the need of sending the change control form to _____ for their review and impact analysis.
    Other departments

15. The planned close-out date will be placed on the _____ by initiator in consultation with all department effected by change.
    Original change control form

QCT-05.14

Assessment for Immunoblotting

YOUR COMPANY NAME

Name: _____ ID No.: _____ Issued by: _____

Designation: _____ Department: _____ Date: _____

1. The immunoblotting is an analytical technique used to detect specific
_____.
   a. Amino acids
   b. Enzymes
   c. Proteins
   d. Carbohydrates

2. This technique relies on the identification of single protein spots via
antigen–antibody-specific reactions from 2D _____.
   a. PAGE
   b. Capillary electrophoresis
   c. HPLC
   d. GC

3. Proteins are typically separated by gel electrophoresis by the length of
the _____ and transferred onto nitrocellulose membranes where
they are detected using antibody-specific target proteins.
   a. Polypeptide structure
   b. DNA structure
   c. Antibodies
   d. Enzymes

4. Detection tags on secondary antibodies are usually enzymes such as
_____ or alkaline phosphatase.
   a. ATP
   b. HRP
   c. ADP
   d. Phosphatase

YOUR COMPANY NAME

Name: _____ ID No.: _____ Issued by: _____

Designation: _____ Department: _____ Date: _____

5. The probed membranes are treated with chemicals which react with the enzymes leading to the generation of light which is known as _____.
   a. 2D electrophoresis
   b. Chemiluminescence
   c. Western blotting
   d. Chromatography

6. Immunoblotting is a good technique to detect _____ even if very small quantities of sample are available.
   a. Carbonyl groups
   b. Proteins
   c. Antibodies
   d. Horse radish peroxidase

7. Immunoblotting can detect as little as _____ amounts of protein, depending on the specificity of the antibodies.
   a. Milligrams
   b. Hectograms
   c. Picograms
   d. Nanograms

8. The generation of electromagnetic radiation as light by the release of energy from a chemical reaction is known as _____.
   a. Radiation
   b. Fluorescence
   c. Chemiluminescence
   d. Ultraviolet radiation

9. Enhanced chemiluminescence or ECL is the technique used for immuno-detection protein _____.
   a. Development
   b. Identification
   c. Extraction
   d. Separation

YOUR COMPANY NAME

Name: _____ ID No.: _____ Issued by: _____

Designation: _____ Department: _____ Date: _____

10. With ECL technique proteins can be detected down to _____
    quantities, which is well below the detection limit for most assay
    systems.
    a. Femto-mole
    b. Millimole
    c. Gram mole
    d. Milligram

11. Light-emitting reactions, which take place by the use of _____,
    are designated electrochemiluminescent reactions.
    a. Synthetic compounds
    b. Electrical current
    c. Living organism
    d. Proteins

12. In chemiluminescent detection methods, _____ membranes are
    first stained to visualize proteins, after which the immunodetection is
    undertaken.
    a. Nitrocellulose
    b. HRP
    c. Polyvinylidene fluoride
    d. HRP-molecule enzyme complex

13. Chemiluminescent detection methods depend on incubation of the
    Western blot with a substrate that will _____ when exposed to
    the reporter on the secondary antibody.
    a. Luminesce
    b. Radiate
    c. Recognize
    d. React

14. Chemiluminescent substrates for HRP are two-component systems con-
    sisting of a stable _____ solution and an enhanced luminol solution.
    a. Protein
    b. Peroxide
    c. Phosphatase
    d. Enzyme

YOUR COMPANY NAME

Name: _____ ID No.: _____ Issued by: _____

Designation: _____ Department: _____ Date: _____

15. During the reaction, the substrate produces a triplet _____ upon
    further oxidation by hydrogen peroxide, which emits light when it decays
    to the singlet carbonyl.
    a. Carbonyl
    b. Hydroxyl
    c. Hydrogen
    d. Peroxide

QCT-05.14.1

Answers to Quiz for Immunoblotting

YOUR COMPANY NAME

Name: _____ ID No.: _____ Issued by: _____

Designation: _____ Department: _____ Date: _____

1. The immunoblotting is an analytical technique used to detect specific _____.

   Proteins

2. This technique relies on the identification of single protein spots via antigen–antibody-specific reactions from 2D _____.
   PAGE

3. Proteins are typically separated by gel electrophoresis by the length of the _____and transferred onto nitrocellulose membranes where they are detected using antibody-specific target proteins.
   Polypeptide structure

4. Detection tags on secondary antibodies are usually enzymes such as _____ or alkaline phosphatase.
   HRP

5. The probed membranes are treated with chemicals which react with the enzymes leading to the generation of light which is known as _____.
   Chemiluminescence

6. Immunoblotting is a good technique to detect _____ even if very small quantities of sample are available.
   Proteins

7. Immunoblotting can detect as little as _____ amounts of protein, depending on the specificity of the antibodies.
   Picograms

YOUR COMPANY NAME

Name: _____ ID No.: _____ Issued by: _____

Designation: _____ Department: _____ Date: _____

8. The generation of electromagnetic radiation as light by the release of energy from a chemical reaction is known as _____.
   Chemiluminescence

9. Enhanced chemiluminescence or ECL is the technique used for immunodetection protein _____.
   Identification

10. With ECL technique proteins can be detected down to _____ quantities, which is well below the detection limit for most assay systems.
    Femto-mole

11. Light-emitting reactions, which take place by the use of _____, are designated electrochemiluminescent reactions.
    Electrical current

12. In chemiluminescent detection methods, _____ membranes are first stained to visualize proteins, after which the immunodetection is undertaken.
    Polyvinylidene fluoride

13. Chemiluminescent detection methods depend on incubation of the Western blot with a substrate that will _____ when exposed to the reporter on the secondary antibody.
    Luminesce

14. Chemiluminescent substrates for HRP are two-component systems consisting of a stable _____ solution and an enhanced luminol solution.
    Peroxide

15. During the reaction, the substrate produces a triplet _____ upon further oxidation by hydrogen peroxide, which emits light when it decays to the singlet carbonyl.
    Carbonyl

QCT-05.15

Assessment for Gel Permeation Chromatography

YOUR COMPANY NAME

Name: _____ ID No.: _____ Issued by: _____

Designation: _____ Department: _____ Date: _____

1. GPC is a widely accepted analytical method used in the separation, purification and characterization of _____.
   a. Bio and synthetic polymers
   b. High molecular weight sugars
   c. Proteins and carbohydrates
   d. Fatty acids

2. In GPC, the separation technique is based on differences in _____ in solution.
   a. Temperature
   b. Molecular size
   c. Solutes
   d. Viscosity

3. Currently, most of the GPC analyses are performed by comparing the _____ of a sample against standards of known molecular weight.
   a. Weight
   b. Solution
   c. Molecular weight
   d. Chromatogram

4. The technique of GPC is based on the size or hydrodynamic volume of the analytes and utilizes a _____ mode of separation, whereas other separation techniques depend upon chemical or physical interactions to separate analytes.
   a. Interactive
   b. Non-interactive
   c. Automatic
   d. Different

YOUR COMPANY NAME

Name: _____ ID No.: _____ Issued by: _____

Designation: _____ Department: _____ Date: _____

5. In the GPC, a stationary phase is used which is composed of a
   _____.
   a. Macromolecular gel
   b. Silica gel
   c. Micro-molecular gel
   d. Cellulose membrane

6. Specific columns used steel cylinder typically 10 mm in diameter and
   _____ in length.
   a. 500–1000 mm
   b. 800 mm
   c. 100 mm
   d. 50 mm

7. The liquid mobile phase is usually water or _____ for biological
   separations mixed with an organic solvent.
   a. Salt
   b. Buffer
   c. Base
   d. Organic acid

8. When columns are created they are packed with _____ with a
   specific pore size so that they are most accurate at separating molecules
   with sizes similar to the pore size.
   a. Porous beads
   b. Silica
   c. Glass
   d. Gel

9. The desired flow rate through the column can be achieved either by
   gravity or by using a _____.
   a. High-pressure pump
   b. Automatic pump
   c. Glass column
   d. Glass beads

YOUR COMPANY NAME

Name: _____ ID No.: _____ Issued by: _____

Designation: _____ Department: _____ Date: _____

10. To separate hydrophilic samples, polar phases are best choice whereas for hydrophobic, _____ phases work most effectively.
    a. Miscible
    b. Non-polar
    c. Buffer
    d. Stationary

11. The SEC separation can be optimized by the selection of appropriate _____ and columns.
    a. Mobile phase
    b. Stationary phase
    c. Detector
    d. Samples

12. Size range of the _____ is one of the important parameters to design an effective SEC separation.
    a. Column
    b. Pores
    c. Molecules
    d. Detector

13. While travelling down the column, the _____ have relatively less number of pores available for them to fit in.
    a. Smaller molecules
    b. Solvent molecules
    c. Larger analyte molecules
    d. Impurities

14. A concentration detector is located at the end of the column to determine the amount of _____ emerging out.
    a. Sample
    b. Solvent
    c. Silica
    d. Pores

YOUR COMPANY NAME

Name: _____ ID No.: _____ Issued by: _____

Designation: _____ Department: _____ Date: _____

15. There is a low chance of loss of analytes since they do not interact chemi-
    cally or physically with _____.
    a. Columns
    b. Each other
    c. Solvent
    d. Solution

16. While travelling through the column, the _____ enter all pores
    larger than their size.
    a. Small-sized molecules
    b. Large-sized molecules
    c. The stationary phase particles
    d. The solvent molecules

17. Since the amount of pores volume available for larger volume will be
    less than those for the small-sized volumes, the larger-sized molecules
    will elute _____.
    a. Later
    b. Quicker
    c. Slowly
    d. After the small-sized molecules

18. GPC provides a more convenient method of determining the
    _____ of polymers.
    a. Structure
    b. Molecular weights
    c. Chemical nature
    d. Physical properties

19. The GPC for polymers requires _____ before using the instru-
    ment so that the dust and particulates may not destroy columns.
    a. Proper cleaning
    b. Filtration
    c. Calibration
    d. Washing

YOUR COMPANY NAME

Name: _____ ID No.: _____ Issued by: _____

Designation: _____ Department: _____ Date: _____

20. A disadvantage of using the pre-filtration is that it may remove _____ samples before loading on the column.
    a. Higher molecular weight
    b. Lower molecular weight
    c. Polymer
    d. Solute

QCT-05.15.1

Answers to Quiz for Gel Permeation Chromatography

YOUR COMPANY NAME

Name: _____ ID No.: _____ Issued by: _____

Designation: _____ Department: _____ Date: _____

1. GPC is a widely accepted analytical method used in the separation, purification and characterization of _____.
   Bio and synthetic polymers

2. In GPC, the separation technique is based on differences in _____ in solution.
   Molecular size

3. Currently, most of the GPC analyses are performed by comparing the _____ of a sample against standards of known molecular weight.
   Molecular weight

4. The technique of GPC is based on the size or hydrodynamic volume of the analytes and utilizes a _____ mode of separation, whereas other separation techniques depend upon chemical or physical interactions to separate analytes.
   Non-interactive

5. In GPC, a stationary phase is used which is composed of a _____.
   Macromolecular gel

6. Specific columns used steel cylinder typically 10 mm in diameter and _____ in length.
   500–1000 mm

YOUR COMPANY NAME

Name: _____ ID No.: _____ Issued by: _____

Designation: _____ Department: _____ Date: _____

7. The liquid mobile phase is usually water or _____ for biological separations mixed with an organic solvent.
   Buffer

8. When columns are created they are packed with _____ with a specific pore size so that they are most accurate at separating molecules with sizes similar to the pore size.
   Porous beads

9. The desired flow rate through the column can be achieved either by gravity or by using a _____.
   High-pressure pump

10. To separate hydrophilic samples, polar phases are best choice whereas for hydrophobic, _____ phases work most effectively.
    Non-polar

11. The SEC separation can be optimized by the selection of appropriate _____ and columns.
    Mobile phase

12. Size range of the _____ is one of the important parameters to design an effective SEC separation.
    Pores

13. While travelling down the column, the _____ have relatively less number of pores available for them to fit in.
    Larger analyte molecules

14. A concentration detector is located at the end of the column to determine the amount of _____ emerging out.
    Sample

15. There is a low chance of loss of analytes since they do not interact chemically or physically with _____.
    Columns

YOUR COMPANY NAME

Name: _____ ID No.: _____ Issued by: _____

Designation: _____ Department: _____ Date: _____

16. While travelling through the column, the _____ enter all pores larger then their size.
    Small-sized molecules

17. Since the amount of pores volume available for larger volume will be less than those for the small-sized volumes, the larger-sized molecules will elute _____.
    Quicker

18. GPC provides a more convenient method of determining the _____ of polymers.
    Molecular weights

19. The GPC for polymers requires _____ before using the instrument so that the dust and particulates may not destroy columns.
    Filtration

20. A disadvantage of using the pre-filtration is that it may remove _____ samples before loading on the column.
    Higher molecular weight

QCT-05.16

Assessment for Electrophoresis

YOUR COMPANY NAME

Name: _____ ID No.: _____ Issued by: _____

Designation: _____ Department: _____ Date: _____

1. The _____ motion of dispersed particles relative to a fluid under the influence of a spatially uniform electric field is known as electrophoresis.
   a. Electrokinetic
   b. Circular
   c. Kinetic
   d. Magnetic

2. Electrophoresis is a technique used in genetic testing to _____ and separate proteins, DNA and RNA.
   a. Produce
   b. Analyse
   c. Synthesize
   d. Mix

3. The interaction of a charged or uncharged molecule normally changes its _____ properties.
   a. Kinetic
   b. Magnetic
   c. Chemical
   d. Electrophoretic

4. Affinity electrophoresis is useful in obtaining both qualitative and _____ information.
   a. Physical
   b. Quantitative
   c. Chemical
   d. Biological

YOUR COMPANY NAME

Name: _____ ID No.: _____ Issued by: _____

Designation: _____ Department: _____ Date: _____

5. The most common type of electrophoresis are gel electrophoresis and
   _____.
   a. Mobility shift electrophoresis
   b. Charge shift electrophoresis
   c. Capillary zone electrophoresis
   d. 2D electrophoresis

6. Gel electrophoresis separates the molecules by _____ and charge
   using different types of gel mediums.
   a. Molecular structure
   b. Molecular weight
   c. Molecular ion
   d. Type of gel used

7. The most commonly used mediums for proteins, DNA and RNA separation are _____ and polyacrylamide.
   a. Agarose
   b. Peptides
   c. Soya broth
   d. EDTA

8. The separation of molecules within a gel is determined by the relative
   size of the _____ formed within the gel.
   a. Molecules
   b. Pores
   c. Polymer
   d. DNA

9. The pore size of a gel is therefore determined by two factors: the total
   amount of acrylamide, and _____.
   a. The amount of cross-linker
   b. The size of proteins
   c. Quantity of gel
   d. Molecular weight

YOUR COMPANY NAME

Name: _____ ID No.: _____ Issued by: _____

Designation: _____ Department: _____ Date: _____

10. If the molecules to be separated are DNA, RNA or oligonucleotides, then the gel is composed of different concentrations of _____ and a cross-linker, producing different sized mesh networks of polyacrylamide.
    a. Agarose
    b. Acrylamide
    c. Proteins
    d. Acid

11. The agarose gels are submerged in buffer used for the separation; that is why the technique is also known as _____.
    a. Capillary electrophoresis
    b. Submarine electrophoresis
    c. 1D electrophoresis
    d. 2D electrophoresis

12. For _____ TAE, TBE and sodium borate (SB) are the most commonly used ones.
    a. 1D electrophoresis
    b. Capillary electrophoresis
    c. Agarose gel electrophoresis
    d. Submarine electrophoresis

13. One dimensional (1D) electrophoresis is also known as _____.
    a. PAGE
    b. Capillary gel electrophoresis
    c. Zone capillary electrophoresis
    d. Agarose gel electrophoresis

14. During the separation phase, the travelling rate for each type of molecule through the medium varies according to its _____ or size.
    a. Electrical charge
    b. Class
    c. Molecular weight
    d. Chemical properties

YOUR COMPANY NAME

Name: _____ ID No.: _____ Issued by: _____

Designation: _____ Department: _____ Date: _____

15. The 2D electrophoresis begins with 1D electrophoresis but then separates the molecules by a second property in a direction _____ from the first.
    a. 80°
    b. 90°
    c. 120°
    d. 180°

16. When the proteins are separated in one dimension, all the molecules lie along a lane but be separated from each other by a property called _____.
    a. Isocratic point
    b. Isoelectric point
    c. Thermal point
    d. Freezing point

17. The applied _____ between the source and destination vials initiates the migration of analytes in capillary electrophoresis.
    a. Magnetic field
    b. Electric field
    c. Charge
    d. Force

18. The velocity of migration of an analyte in CE depends upon the rate of _____ flow of the buffer solution.
    a. Electro-osmotic
    b. Particles
    c. Ionic
    d. Electrolytic

19. During the migration phase, separation of electrolytes takes place according to their _____.
    a. Ionic charge
    b. Electrophoretic mobility
    c. Molecular weight
    d. Magnetic field

YOUR COMPANY NAME

Name: _____ ID No.: _____ Issued by: _____

Designation: _____ Department: _____ Date: _____

20. Typically, the electro-osmotic flow is directed towards the
    _____.
    a. Anode
    b. Cathode
    c. Destination vial
    d. Buffer solution

QCT-05.16.1

Answers to Quiz for Electrophoresis

YOUR COMPANY NAME

Name: _____ ID No.: _____ Issued by: _____

Designation: _____ Department: _____ Date: _____

1. The _____ motion of dispersed particles relative to a fluid under the influence of a spatially uniform electric field is known as electrophoresis.
   Electrokinetic

2. Electrophoresis is a technique used in genetic testing to _____ and separate proteins, DNA and RNA.
   Analyse

3. The interaction of a charged or uncharged molecule normally changes its _____ properties.
   Electrophoretic

4. Affinity electrophoresis is useful in obtaining both qualitative and _____ information.
   Quantitative

5. The most common type of electrophoresis are gel electrophoresis and _____.
   Capillary zone electrophoresis

6. Gel electrophoresis separates the molecules by _____ and charge using different types of gel mediums.
   Molecular weight

7. The most commonly used mediums for proteins: DNA and RNA separation are _____ and polyacrylamide.
   Agarose

YOUR COMPANY NAME

Name: _____ ID No.: _____ Issued by: _____

Designation: _____ Department: _____ Date: _____

8. The separation of molecules within a gel is determined by the relative size of the _____ formed within the gel.
   Pores

9. The pore size of a gel is therefore determined by two factors: the total amount of acrylamide, and _____
   The amount of cross-linker

10. If the molecules to be separated are DNA, RNA or oligonucleotides, then the gel is composed of different concentrations of _____ and a cross-linker, producing different sized mesh networks of polyacrylamide.
    Acrylamide

11. The agarose gels are submerged in buffer used for the separation; that is why the technique is also known as _____ .
    Submarine-electrophoresis

12. For _____ TAE, TBE and sodium borate (SB) are the most commonly used ones.
    Agarose gel electrophoresis

13. One-dimensional (1D) electrophoresis is also known as _____ .
    PAGE

14. During the separation phase, the travelling rate for each type of molecule through the medium varies according to its _____ or size.
    Electrical charge

15. The 2D electrophoresis begins with 1D electrophoresis but then separates the molecules by a second property in a direction _____ from the first.
    90°

16. When the proteins are separated in one dimension, all the molecules lie along a lane but be separated from each other by a property called

    _____ .

    Isoelectric point

YOUR COMPANY NAME

Name: _____ ID No.: _____ Issued by: _____

Designation: _____ Department: _____ Date: _____

17. The applied _____ between the source and destination vials initiates the migration of analytes in CE.
    Electric field

18. The velocity of migration of an analyte in CE depends upon the rate of _____ flow of the buffer solution.
    Electro osmotic

19. During the migration phase, separation of electrolytes takes place according to their _____.
    Electrophoretic mobility

20. Typically, the electro-osmotic flow is directed towards the _____.
    Cathode

QCT-05.17

Assessment for Ion-Exchange Chromatography

YOUR COMPANY NAME

Name: _____ ID No.: _____ Issued by: _____

Designation: _____ Department: _____ Date: _____

1. IEC is a process that allows the separation of ions and polar molecules based on charge _____.
   a. Repulsions
   b. Attractions
   c. Interactions
   d. Reactions

2. In biochemistry, IEC is widely used to separate _____ charged molecules.
   a. Unreacted
   b. Charged
   c. Neutral
   d. Protein

3. IEC can also be used for the separation of peptides and _____.
   a. Oligonucleotides
   b. Polypeptides
   c. Halides
   d. Polysaccharides

4. Ion-exchange resin consists of an insoluble _____ with charge groups covalently attached.
   a. Molecule
   b. Matrix
   c. Salt
   d. Material

YOUR COMPANY NAME

Name: _____ ID No.: _____ Issued by: _____

Designation: _____ Department: _____ Date: _____

5. The matrix may be based on inorganic compounds, synthetic resins or
   _____.
   a. Polysaccharides
   b. Peptides
   c. Buffer solution
   d. Positive ions

6. The adsorption of the molecules to the _____ is driven by the
   ionic interaction between the two moieties and binding capacities are
   generally quite high.
   a. Resin
   b. Mobile phase
   c. Solid support
   d. Column

7. The number and location of the _____ on the molecule and solid
   support determine the strength of the interaction.
   a. Groups
   b. Charges
   c. Protein molecules
   d. Negative ions

8. By increasing the salt concentration the molecules with the _____
   ionic interactions are disrupted first and elute earlier in the salt
   gradient.
   a. Strongest
   b. Weakest
   c. Equal
   d. Little

9. Separation of proteins through IEC occurs according to their net charges
   which is dependent on the _____ of the mobile phase.
   a. Nature
   b. Composition
   c. Strength
   d. Charge

YOUR COMPANY NAME

Name: _____ ID No.: _____ Issued by: _____

Designation: _____ Department: _____ Date: _____

10. Increase in the _____ of the mobile phase buffer results in the decrease in positive charge of the molecule by becoming less protonated.
    a. Viscosity
    b. pH
    c. Concentration
    d. Density

11. Matrices have capacity to bind from 10 to 100 mg of _____ per mL.
    a. Protein
    b. Slurry
    c. Resin
    d. Buffer

12. The anion exchange chromatography is performed using _____ at pHs between 7 and 10.
    a. Acids
    b. Bases
    c. Buffers
    d. Salt

13. The salt in the solution competes for binding to the immobilized matrix and releases the _____ from its bound state at a given concentration.
    a. Protein
    b. Charges
    c. Resin
    d. Protons

14. Characteristically, CEC is performed with buffers at pHs between 4 and _____.
    a. 8
    b. 6
    c. 7
    d. 3

YOUR COMPANY NAME

Name: _____ ID No.: _____ Issued by: _____

Designation: _____ Department: _____ Date: _____

15. The CEC is run on gradient starting from a solution containing the buffer only to a solution containing the buffer with 1 M _____
    a. NaCl
    b. NaBr
    c. Sulphuric acid
    d. HCl

QCT-05.17.1

Answers to Quiz for Ion-Exchange Chromatography

YOUR COMPANY NAME

Name: _____ ID No.: _____ Issued by: _____

Designation: _____ Department: _____ Date: _____

1. IEC is a process that allows the separation of ions and polar molecules based on charge _____.
   Interactions

2. In biochemistry, IEC is widely used to separate _____ molecules.
   Charged

3. IEC can also be used for the separation of peptides and _____.
   Oligonucleotides

4. Ion-exchange resin consists of an insoluble _____ with charge groups covalently attached.
   Matrix

5. The matrix may be based on inorganic compounds, synthetic resins or _____.
   Polysaccharides

6. The adsorption of the molecules to the _____ is driven by the ionic interaction between the two moieties and binding capacities are generally quite high.
   Resin

7. The number and location of the _____ on the molecule and solid support determine the strength of the interaction.
   Charges

YOUR COMPANY NAME

Name: _____ ID No.: _____ Issued by: _____

Designation: _____ Department: _____ Date: _____

8. By increasing the salt concentration the molecules with the _____
   ionic interactions are disrupted first and elute earlier in the salt gradient.
   Weakest

9. Separation of proteins through IEC occurs according to their net charges
   which is dependent on the _____ of the mobile phase.
   Composition

10. Increase in the _____ of the mobile phase buffer results in the
    decrease in positive charge of the molecule by becoming less
    protonated.
    pH

11. Matrices have capacity to bind from 10 to 100 mg of _____
    per mL.
    Protein

12. The anion exchange chromatography is performed using _____
    at pH between 7 and 10.
    Buffers

13. The salt in the solution competes for binding to the immobilized matrix
    and releases the _____ from its bound state at a given
    concentration.
    Protein

14. Characteristically, CEC is performed with buffers at pHs between 4 and
    _____.
    7

15. The CEC is run on gradient starting from a solution containing the buf-
    fer only to a solution containing the buffer with 1 M _____.
    NaCl

QCT-06

Training Log

QCT-06.1

General Introduction Training Log

YOUR COMPANY NAME

Name: _____ ID No.: _____ Issued by: _____

Designation: _____ Department: _____ Date: _____

GENERAL INTRODUCTION OF COMPANY AND DEPARTMENT

Objectives	Date Completed	Trainee Signature	Departmental Manager	Remarks
Have an appreciation of the company's products, organization and place in industry.				
Understand his/her function within the department.				
Understand the work of the department and what its aims and objectives are.				
Understand the departmental organization and lines of authority.				
Understand his/her department's relationship with the rest of the company.				

QCT-06.2

Good Housekeeping and Good Laboratory Practice

YOUR COMPANY NAME

Name: _____ ID No.: _____ Issued by: _____

Designation: _____ Department: _____ Date: _____

GOOD HOUSEKEEPING SAFETY AND GLP

TRAINING LOG PART 2

Name: _____

Department: _____

Designation: _____

Previous Experience: _____

Objectives
Date
Trainee
Approved
Remarks

1. Conversant with the laboratory layout including devices such as fire extinguishers and hazards of the gas and vacuum.
2. Aware of the responsibilities under company safety policy.
3. Aware of the need for personal hygiene and the eating and smoking rule.
4. Aware of the procedure for accident and illness.
5. Have an understanding of the types.
6. Knowing the general chemical hazards of the laboratory and the five golden rules.
7. Aware of the correct waste disposal systems.
8. Aware of the danger of emissions within the laboratory.

YOUR COMPANY NAME

Name: _____ ID No.: _____ Issued by: _____

Designation: _____ Department: _____ Date: _____

9. Aware of the rules covering electrical equipment.
10. Aware of the correct methods of glass equipment assembly and the correct disposal of glass and other sharp objects.
11. Aware of the rules on non-authorized work.
12. Aware of the nine golden rules of the microbiological control laboratory.
13. Understand the importance of analytical work and of following methods correctly.
14. Understand the importance of no alterations or shortcuts to methods.
15. Understand where methods are derived from.
16. Know where to go for assistance/help if in doubt.
17. Know what an SOP is and its importance.
18. Know the difference in the degrees of accuracy of methods.
19. Know the importance of expiry dates of reagents.
20. Know how to use the laboratory.
21. Know the consequences.
22. Know the importance of raw data storage.
23. Know the limitations of some analytical methods.
24. Know the difference between accuracy and precision.
25. Know where to find reference books in the laboratory.
26. Know what other sources of information are available.
27. Know the responsibility of the position held.

QCT-06.3

Sampling Procedure Training Log

YOUR COMPANY NAME

Name: _____ ID No.: _____ Issued by: _____

Designation: _____ Department: _____ Date: _____

TRAINING OF SAMPLING PROCEDURE

Name: _____
Department: _____
Designation: _____
Previous Experience: _____

Objectives
Date
Trainee
Approved
Remarks
Hours

COMPLETED

Signature
SPENT HOURS

1. Understand the potential hazards involved and the importance of representative sampling in analytical work.
2. Are able to apply basic sampling techniques.
3. Are able to render a sample uniform, prior to testing using appropriate methods.
4. Understand the departmental requirements.
5. Understand your department's relationship with the rest of the company.
6. Understand the grievance and disciplinary procedures in use.
7. Understand the departmental training policy, regarding absence, sickness and holidays.
8. Are conversant with all items of general welfare within the company.

QCT-06.4

Chemical Testing Training Log

YOUR COMPANY NAME

Name: _____ ID No.: _____ Issued by: _____

Designation: _____ Department: _____ Date: _____

TRAINING OF CHEMICAL TESTING

Objectives	Date Completed	Trainee	Approved Yes/No	Remarks
Weighing				
1. Can weigh to an appropriate accuracy.				
2. Understands the different types of balance available and when each should be used.				
3. Can use each balance according to its SOP.				
4. Understands the potential sources of error in weighing.				
5. Assessment.				
Volumetric Techniques				
1. Measure to appropriate accuracy.				
2. Knows how and when to use appropriate graduated and non-graduated glassware.				
3. Can use volumetric apparatus correctly (including pipettes, burettes, volumetric flasks, etc.).				
4. Can titrate to a satisfactory accuracy.				
5. Assessment.				
Temperature Measurement and Control				
1. Able to use the thermometers correctly and safely.				
2. Know when to use standardized and non-standardized thermometers.				
3. Know what heating and cooling sources are available and when and how to use them, bearing in mind potential hazards.				
4. Can determine the melting point of a suitable sample to the required accuracy.				
5. Assessment.				

YOUR COMPANY NAME

Name: _____ ID No.: _____ Issued by: _____

Designation: _____ Department: _____ Date: _____

Objectives	Date Completed	Trainee	Approved Yes/No	Remarks
Mechanical Methods of Separation				
1. Know how to use the different types of filtration methods in the laboratory.				
2. Understand the appropriate cleaning procedures and the potential hazards involved in solvent extractions using separating funnels.				
3. Can carry out a simple quantitative solvent extraction exercise.				
4. Can use a centrifuge in a safe and efficient manner.				
5. Assessment.				
Limit Test				
1. Understand the use and limitations of limit test.				
2. Understand the basic principles and procedures used and the differences between EP, BP and USP limits.				
3. Aware of any potential hazards.				
4. Can carry out limit tests correctly according to the appropriate methods.				
5. Assessment				
5.1. Chloride				
5.2. Sulphate				
5.3. Iron				
5.4. Heavy metals (or lead)				
5.5. Sulphated ash				
5.6. Loss on drying				
Weight per mL/Density				
1. Understand the different ways in which the wt/mL of a liquid can be determined and the factors affecting the results.				
2. Understand and know how to look for potential hazards.				
3. Can carry out the wt/mL determination of a liquid correctly according to the appropriate method or SOP.				
4. Assessment.				

YOUR COMPANY NAME

Name: _____ ID No.: _____ Issued by: _____

Designation: _____ Department: _____ Date: _____

Objectives	Date Completed	Trainee	Approved Yes/No	Remarks
Weight per mL/Density 1. Understand how to determine the apparent density of a solid according to the appropriate method and SOP. 2. Understand and know how to look for potential hazards. 3. Assessment.				
Physical Observation 1. Understand the possible hazards involved with some compounds—that is, toxic materials. 2. Understand the importance of these tests with regard to approval of material, assessment of deterioration, and so on. 3. Know how to use any relevant procedures for determining colour, clarity, and so on, according to appropriate methods or SOPs. 4. Can accurately report the physical characteristics of given materials.				
Testing to Specification/Practical Work 1. Able to test samples or carry out his/her work efficiently without deviation from established procedures and with minimum guidance.				
Chromatographic Techniques for TLC, GC, and HPLC methods 1. Understand the basic principles and procedures used in chromatographic separations and determination. 2. Understand and know how to look for potential hazards. 3. Understand the limitations of the methods. 4. Can recognize common faults leading to poor chromatograms and know how to deal with them. 5. Can use the appropriate departmental equipment according to SOPs or manufacturer's instructions.				

YOUR COMPANY NAME

Name: _____ ID No.: _____ Issued by: _____

Designation: _____ Department: _____ Date: _____

Objectives	Date Completed	Trainee	Approved Yes/No	Remarks
6. Can carry out simple chromatographic separations and determinations to achieve the required degree of accuracy.				
7. Assessment				
7.1. TLC				
7.2. HPLC				
7.3. GC				
Spectroscopic Techniques				
1. For visible, UV, IR, AAS, and Fe (II) spectroscopy methods.				
2. Understand the basic principles and procedures used.				
3. Understand and know how to look for potential hazards.				
4. Understand the limitations of the methods.				
5. Can recognize common faults leading to poor spectra or wrong results and how to deal with them.				
6. Can determine the IR spectra of suitable materials using appropriate sample preparation techniques.				
7. Can carry out a simple AAS exercise to the required accuracy.				
8. Assessment				
8.1. Calorimetric				
8.2. UV absorption				
8.3. Infrared spectrum				
8.4. AAS				
Electrochemical Techniques				
1. For pH, ISE, potentiometric, biamperometric and automatic titrations and polarography.				
2. Understand the basic principles and procedures used.				
3. Understand and know how to look for potential hazards.				
4. Understand the limitations of the methods.				
5. Can recognize common faults leading to incorrect results and know how to check equipment before use.				

YOUR COMPANY NAME

Name: _____ ID No.: _____ Issued by: _____

Designation: _____ Department: _____ Date: _____

Objectives	Date Completed	Trainee	Approved Yes/No	Remarks
Miscellaneous Techniques				
For colorimetric, particle size and viscometry:				
1. Understand the basic principles and procedures used.				
2. Understand and know how to look for potential hazards.				
3. Understand the limitations of the methods.				
4. Can recognize common faults leading to incorrect results and know how to check equipment before use.				
5. Can carry the appropriate Departmental instrumentation according to the relevant SOPs.				
6. Assessment				
6.1. Polarimetric				
6.2. Particle size				
6.3. Viscometry				
Other Analytical Techniques				
For disintegration and dissolution:				
1. Understand the basic principles and procedures used.				
2. Understand and know how to look for potential hazards.				
3. Understand the limitations of the methods.				
4. Demonstrate the ability to recognize common faults leading to incorrect results and know how to check equipment prior to use.				
5. Must complete the relevant sections of any departmental training instructions prior to starting normal work for any other techniques.				

QCT-06.5

Training Log for Microbiology

YOUR COMPANY NAME

Name: _____ ID No.: _____ Issued by: _____

Designation: _____ Department: _____ Date: _____

Objectives	Date Completed	Trainee	Approved	Remarks
1. Use of Balance and Volumetric Techniques Weigh accurately a clean weighing bottle. Add 10 mL water from a 10-mL cylinder and reweigh. Calculate the volume of water added from volume = Weight of water where w is the wt mL of water at RT. Repeat the exercise: 1. 10 mL water measured from a 50-mL cylinder 2. 10 mL water measured from a 10-mL graduated pipette 3. 10 mL water measured from a 50-mL burette 4. 3×10 mL water measured from a 10-mL one mark pipette of known calibration Assessment: The results obtain for the 3×10 mL pipettings from the one mark pipette should have a maximum spread of 0.02 mL and the mean of the three should be 10.00 + 0.02 mL.				
2. Temperature Measurement and Control 1. The trainee should be able to use correctly, according to relevant SOPs, all forms of heating and cooling used within the laboratory—that is, burners, ovens, steam or water baths, ice baths, and so on.				

YOUR COMPANY NAME

Name: _____ ID No.: _____ Issued by: _____

Designation: _____ Department: _____ Date: _____

Objectives	Date Completed	Trainee	Approved	Remarks
2. The trainee should carry out at least two determinations of the melting point or melting range of substance readily reduced to a powder according to appropriate methods. 3. Criteria for acceptance: The trainee should have used the apparatus correctly. The melting points or ranges obtained by the trainee should be as expected. If the trainee's results are not as expected, the trainer should decide whether the tests need to be repeated, if necessary, after a further period of training.				
3. Media Preparation 1. The trainee should prepare any two types of liquid media and any two types of solid media. 2. Criteria for acceptance: The appearance, that is, colour, clarity, solidification, if appropriate, should all be as given in the manufacturer's guidelines. 3. The appropriate organism(s) should be cultured on/in the media and growth and appearance should be as in the manufacturer's guidelines.				
4. Glassware Preparation Not applicable. However, the trainee should spend at least a week preparing and washing all forms of glassware.				
5. Aseptic Technique Not applicable. However, the acceptability of the trainee's technique will become apparent during the normal days as controls are used in various tests to check for contamination and aseptic procedures.				

YOUR COMPANY NAME

Name: _____ ID No.: _____ Issued by: _____

Designation: _____ Department: _____ Date: _____

Objectives	Date Completed	Trainee	Approved	Remarks

6. Autoclaves
  1. The trainee should carry out calibration of the autoclaves in accordance with instructions and SOPs
  2. Criteria for acceptance: providing the autoclave is functioning properly, all calibration checks should be in accordance with instructions and SOPs				

7. Laminar Flow/Safety Cabinets Not applicable.				

8. Testing to Specification/ Practical Work
An experienced analyst should test the practical work or samples tested by the trainee. In all cases, the results obtained by the trainee should have been within the accuracy and precision of the methods carried out and similar to those obtained by an experienced analyst.
  If the trainee's results do not meet those requirements, the trainer should decide whether any tests need repeating and, if necessary, carry out further training as required.
  The trainee should not be allowed to carry out actual work until the trainer is satisfied that he/she has reached an acceptable standard.				

9. Microbiological Assays
  1. The trainee should first carry out an assay using approved method.
 	
  The trainer should assess the following:
 	
  Assay plates or trays have marked correctly.
  2. The required information has been entered into appropriate books and that computer printouts also have this information.
  3. Accuracy of assay compared to previous assay on the same lot of product.				

YOUR COMPANY NAME

Name: _____ ID No.: _____ Issued by: _____

Designation: _____ Department: _____ Date: _____

Objectives	Date Completed	Trainee	Approved	Remarks
3.1 All check samples, if necessary, are within limits.				
3.2 The raw data are within certain acceptable limits so as to give appropriate valid assays.				
Criteria for acceptance:				
1. The assay has been carried out in accordance with the principles given in the appropriate SOP, ensuring correct marking and identification of assay plates and trays.				
2. The assay in the required range of previous assays and the check samples are within the required control limits.				
3. If the trainee's results are not within these requirements, the trainer should decide whether the exercise should be repeated, if necessary, after a further period of training.				
10. pH Measurement				
1. The trainee should prepare a suitable solution and measure its pH according to the relevant SOPs.				
2. An experienced analyst should have previously analysed all samples used.				

QCT-07

Analytical Method Validation Master Plan

Product Development

Written by **Quality Control Manager** _____	**Signature & Date**

Reviewed by **Research and Development Manager** _____	**Signature & Date**

Approved by **Quality Assurance Director** _____	**Signature & Date**

PURPOSE

The purpose of this Validation Master Plan is to describe the strategy for analytical methods validation programme for existing and new products in ABC Pharmaceutical Industries. The Validation Plan will outline the set of activities customized to provide validation programs that ensure compliance with industry standards and regulations.

This Validation Master Plan further describes the approach for use in the development of protocols and procedures for method validation. It outlines the validation requirements to ensure compliance with regulatory policies.

- The plan shall describe the methods to be validated and the general methodology to be used for validation.
- It will outline the validation philosophy and roles and responsibilities of other departments involved.
- It will serve as a liaison to communicate with regulatory agencies.
- It will serve as a guideline to those administering and performing method validation activities.

INTRODUCTION

Validated analytical test methods are required by GMP regulations for products that have been authorized for sale and almost certainly for late-stage trial clinical material. Analytical methods development and validation play important roles in the discovery, development and manufacture of pharmaceuticals. Methods used during the pre-clinical phase of drug development under good QCT-07.5 practice regulations may also require validation prior to their implementation.

QC laboratories need to ensure the identity, purity, potency and performance of drug products, and use the official test methods that result from these processes.

Analytical methods validation can be defined as the measures taken to prove that the analytical methods employed for a specific test is suitable for its intended use, consistently perform as expected and produce results that consistently meet predetermined specifications.

Method validation has received considerable attention from industrial committees and regulatory agencies and is applied to all analytical procedures used for all dosage forms of products in pharmaceutical industries.

The Method Validation Master Plan will ensure that the testing procedures/methods meet the compliance requirements outlined in the cGMP and current Good Laboratory Practice (cGLP)—QCT-7.5. Specifically, it ensures that ABC Pharmaceutical Industries will meet the relevant requirements for:

a. United States Food and Drug Administration (FDA)
b. European Pharmacopoeia (EP)

When the items detailed in the Methods Validation Master Plan are completed, the accuracy, reliability and consistency of the analytical methods, instruments and skills of analysts to test products to levels that are below concern will be documented and will ensure reproducibility of the test procedures and thereby constant product quality.

The process of analytical method's validation should demonstrate that the method is fit for its purpose. The validation should follow a plan that includes the scope of the method, the method performance characteristics and acceptance limits. Parameters usually examined in the validation process are limits of detection and quantitation, accuracy, precision, selectivity/specificity, linearity, range and ruggedness. A validation report should be generated with all experimental conditions and the complete statistics. When "standard" methods are used in the QCT-07.5, their scope should be in line with the scope of the laboratories' method requirements and the suitability of the entire analytical system in the specific QCT-07.5's environment should be verified for the method.

Methods need to be validated or revalidated

a. Before their introduction into routine use
b. Whenever the conditions change for which the method has been validated, for example, instrument with different characteristics
c. Whenever the method is changed, and the change is outside the original scope of the method

SCOPE AND APPROACH

This Validation Master Plan covers the validation of analytical methods used at the ABC Pharmaceutical Industries. The scope of this plan addresses the validation requirements to prove the accuracy of test methods to ensure precision of analytical results to meet the pre-determined limits.

The Analytical Validation Master Plan will ensure that the analyses approach of ABC Pharmaceutical Industries is consistent with accepted industry practices and published health-based guidelines of the FDA, and European Regulatory Agencies.

The approach in method validation is to perform a series of experiments designed to estimate certain types of analytical errors, for example, a linearity experiment to determine reportable range, a replication experiment to estimate imprecision or random error, a comparison of methods experiment to estimate inaccuracy or systematic error, or interference, recovery experiments to specifically estimate constant and proportional systematic errors (analytical specificity), and a detection limit experiment to characterize analytical sensitivity.

Matrix for all products manufactured at the ABC Pharmaceutical Industries facility is presented in Table 7.1.

The information contained in this plan shall be reviewed annually to ensure that it remains current with existing STMs, instruments and policies. All previous versions of the Analytical Validation Master Plan shall be kept on file for reference.

The scope of the Method Validation Master Plan also includes the different types of equipment and the locations where the method will be run.

TABLE 7.1
Matrix for Products Manufactured at ABC Pharmaceutical Industries

Tablets

Thidoxine
Thiamine 100 mg
Cyanocobalamine 200 mg
Paracetamol 500 mg
Albendazole 400 mg; 800 mg
Amiodarone 200 mg
Bromocryptin 2.5 mg
Ketotifen fumarate 1 mg; 2 mg
Oxybuprocaine Lozenges
Tyrothricin 4.0 mg; 24 mg
Betamethasone 0.5 mg; 5 mg
Salbutamol 4 mg; 16 mg
Captopril 50 mg
Propranolol 40 mg
Cetrizine 10 mg
Chlorpheniramine
Cimetidin 400 mg
Ciprofloxacin 500 mg F/C
Clarithromycin 500 mg
Diclofenac 50 mg
Metformin 100 mg F/C
Diazepam 5 mg
Dimenhydrinate
Erythromycin 500 mg
Dextromethorphan
Famotidine 40 mg
Carbamazepine 200 mg
Antiflu tablets
Folic acid 5 mg
Gliclazide 80 mg
Prednisolone
Promethasone 25 mg F/C
Indapamide 2.5 mg F/C
Diphenoxylate
Atropine 0.025 mg; 0.3 mg
Levofloxacin F/C
Paracetamol 500 mg
Aspirin 81 mg E/C
Aspirin 300 mg E/C
Attapulgite
Lamotrigine 100 mg
Sennosides 12 mg; 72 mg

TABLE 7.1   (continued)

Matrix for Products Manufactured at ABC Pharmaceutical Industries

Bisacodyl 5 mg

Bezafibrate 200 mg

Lomefloxacin 400 mg

Acyclovir 800 mg

Loratadine 10 mg

Mebendazole 100 mg

Methyldopa 250 mg F/C

Glibenclamide

Multivitamin M

Nicotinamide 15 mg; 45 mg/day

Bromhexine 8 mg

Ambroxol 30 mg

Orphenadrine

Enalapril 20 mg

Metronidazole 500 mg

Mebendazole 100 mg 200 mg

Ibuprofen 600 mg

Metoclopramide 10 mg

Pyridoxine 40 mg

Ranitidine 300 mg F/C

Clarithromycin 500

Simethicone tablets

Furosemide 40 mg

Hyoscine butyl S/C

Pseudoephedrine

Simvastatin 20 mg

Ascorbic acid

Tamoxifen 10 mg

Capsules

Indomethacin 25 mg

Tetracycline 250 mg

Oxytetracycline HCl

Carbinoxamine 10 mg

Fluoxetine 20 mg

Azithromycin 250 mg

Syrup

Paracetamol

Diphenhydramine

Salbutamol

B complex, Vitamin B1, B2, B6 and B12

Ephedrine

Chlorpheniramine maleate 8 mg

continued

TABLE 7.1   (continued)

Matrix for Products Manufactured at ABC Pharmaceutical Industries

Antiflu Paracetamol

Promethazine HCl

Pheniramine

Vitamins A and B complex

Valproate sodium

Furosemide

Bromhexine

Clobutinol HCl

Orciprenaline sulphate

Metoclopramide

Chlorpheniramine glyceryl guaiacolate

Triprolidine HCl

Pseudoephedrine HCl

Dextromethorphan 30 mg

Hyoscine-N-butylbromide

Ketotifen fumarate 2 mg

Cetirizine HCl

Iron sulphate

Loratadine 10 mg

Ambroxol HCl 10 mg

Furosemide 40 mg

Oxybuprocaine solution

Chlorhexidine mouthwash

Suspension

Kaolin

Al–Mg hydroxide

Cotrimoxazole

Simethicone

Ibuprofen

Paracetamol

Carbamazepine

Al–Mg hydroxide/Simethicone

Metronidazole 125 mg

Mebendazole

Nystatin

Albendazole

Drops

Oxymetazoline 0.05%

Paracetamol 300 mg/day

Vitamins A and D

Pipenzolate methyl bromide

Multivitamins

TABLE 7.1   (continued)
Matrix for Products Manufactured at ABC Pharmaceutical Industries
Metoclopramide

Ointment

Betamethasone valerate
Gentamicin sulphate
Nystatin
Neomycin sulphate
Gramicidin
Triamcinolone acetonide
Hydrocortisone
Cinchocaine ointment
Fusidic acid
Acyclovir
Tribenoside/lidocaine
Fluticasone propionate
Clobetasol propionate
Propionate 0.05%

Injectables

Vitamin B1, B6 and B12
Bacitracin
Cimetidine
Diclofenac
Cyanocobalamine
Calcitriol 1 mcg/mL
Amikacin 500 mg/2 mL
Metoclopramide
Ranitidine 50 mg/2 mL
Omeprazole 40 mg
Hyoscine-*N*-butyl bromide 20 mg/1 mL
Vancomycin 0.5 g

METHOD VALIDATION TEAM RESPONSIBILITIES

This Master Plan presents a medium in which the departments concerned with completing the analytical validation can mutually ensure regulatory compliance. The management (and/or designate) of product development QCT-07.5, QC (Chemical and Microbiology) and QA will

a. Agree on the requirements of the Validation Master Plan prior to implementation
b. Discuss/determine the validation approach for completing each segment of the Validation Master Plan
c. Direct the integration and maintenance of the Validation Master Plan

SPECIFIC RESPONSIBILITIES

Specific responsibilities of groups and individuals supporting the analytical methods validation are the following:

RESEARCH AND DEVELOPMENT

a. Develop analytical methods.
b. Write method validation protocols and reports.
c. Review and approve all validation protocols prior to implementation.
d. Execute the protocols with appropriate departments.
e. Review with QC and QA, the development of the validation protocols and the final reports.
f. Approve validation reports merge with the above point.
g. Co-develop an ongoing monitoring program (wherever applicable) to demonstrate that the processes are being maintained under control.
h. Review results and assemble test data into report format for approval.
i. Provide documented training for all personnel responsible for method validation.
j. Ensure that all critical instruments used in method validation are calibrated and qualified.

QC DEPARTMENT

a. Review protocols and reports to conformance with GLPs and internal procedures.
b. Support/advise on the development and updating of all relevant SOPs and documentation.
c. Provide analytical technical support, wherever required.
d. Notify departments of test results.
e. Provide documented training for all personnel responsible for sample testing.

QA DEPARTMENT

a. Review protocols and reports to conformance with GLPs and internal procedures.
b. Support/advise on the development and updating of all relevant SOPs and documentation.

METHOD VALIDATION STRATEGIES

In ABC Pharmaceutical Industries, the test methods were developed on HPLC. These test methods are being validated as per this master plan.

The validity of a specific method should be demonstrated in the SOP (QCT-123) experiments using samples or standards that are similar.

To accomplish the validation of analytical methods a protocol will be developed which will further address the following items:

1. The application, purpose and scope of the method
2. Performance parameters and acceptance criteria
3. Experiments that will be conducted to perform validation
4. Define criteria for re-validation

Further to development of validation protocol, the following actions will be taken:

1. Verify relevant performance characteristics of equipment.
2. Check availability of qualifying materials, for example, standards and reagents.
3. Perform pre-validation experiments.
4. Adjust method parameters or/and acceptance criteria if necessary.
5. Perform full internal (and external) validation experiments.
6. Develop SOPs for executing the method in the routine analysis.
7. Define type and frequency of system suitability tests.
8. QC checks for the routine analysis.
9. Document validation experiments and results in the validation report.

The optimal sequence of validation experiments, in general, will be as follows:

a. Selectivity of standards (optimizing separation and detection of standard mixtures)
b. Precision of retention times and peak areas
c. Linearity, limit of quantitation, limit of detection and range
d. Selectivity with real samples
e. Trueness/accuracy, at different concentrations
f. Ruggedness

NEW PRODUCTS, METHODS AND INSTRUMENTS

The introduction of any new product, method and/or equipment must proceed through ABC Pharmaceutical Industries change control procedure ABC-000. All requirements will be attached to the relevant change control forms.

Before the introduction of any new product or instrument to the QCT-123, an evaluation is to be made using the following criteria:

a. Qualification of the instrument
b. Development of test methods
c. Validation/verification of methods

If a new instrument is included in the QCT-123, assessment will be done to ensure if the existing method will be applicable on the new instrument or a revalidation is required.

Similarly, in case of a new product, the test methods will be developed and consequently validated as per the Master Validation Plan.

REVALIDATION

A revalidation is necessary whenever a method is changed and the new parameter is outside the operating range. If, for example, the operating range of the column temperature has been specified to be between 30°C and 40°C, the method will be revalidated if, for whatever reason, the new operating parameter has been selected as beyond 40°C.

Revalidation is also required if the sample matrix changes and if the instrument type changes, for example, if a brand with significantly different instrument characteristics is used. Similarly, a revalidation will be performed, if an HPLC method has been developed and validated on a pump with a delay volume of 5 mL and the new pump has a different volume.

Part or full revalidation may also be considered if system suitability tests or the results of QC sample analysis are out of preset acceptance criteria and the source of the error cannot be tracked back to instruments or anything else.

PROTOCOL DEVELOPMENT PHASE

A method validation protocol will be developed for each product identified from the matrix incorporating the guidelines and requirements.

As is the case with all method validations, a preliminary assessment is required prior to preparing the protocol.

A typical validation protocol format should include:

1. Approval page for signatures: The signature page indicates persons required to review, approve and sign off the protocol.
2. Title: The title of the method clearly describes the type of methods to identify it from other similar methods. Along with the title, there will be an assigned, unique protocol number.
3. Purpose: The purpose of the protocol is to document that the method consistently, reliably and reproducibly provides the expected result.
4. Introduction: The introduction needs to be clearly written for the individuals responsible for executing the protocol, as well as for those who are responsible for reviewing, approving and auditing the studies.
5. Responsibilities: In this section, participants and their assigned functions will be described. This will include the persons or titles of the individuals who will be responsible for reviewing the protocol. In case of outside consultant's involvement, their names will also be listed.

6. Pre-qualification requirements: This section will identify the equipment, material, reference standards, QC material, supporting methods and technician training that may be required to be completed prior to beginning the specific method validation.
7. Materials and equipment: The manufacturer, model and device number will be listed for all equipments. Materials will be described by their description, manufacturer, catalogue number, containers, and so on.
8. Procedure outline with test functions and acceptance criteria: The procedure will be described in sections corresponding to the test functions as per the following format:
    i. Description
    ii. Purpose
    iii. Acceptance criteria
    iv. Procedure
9. Test report with conclusions: The test report will contain subsections that address each of the parameters tested individually. In each subsection, the results will be briefly summarized with a conclusion drawn as to whether the acceptance criteria for the parameter were met.
10. Method validation parameters: The parameters for validation of analytical methods are summarized in the following paragraphs and will be addressed in the validation protocols for the method validation.
    1. Selectivity and specificity
    2. Precision and reproducibility
    3. Repeatability
    4. Intermediate precision
    5. Accuracy
    6. Trueness
    7. Bias linearity
    8. Range
    9. Limit of detection
    10. Limit of quantitation
    11. Robustness
    12. Ruggedness

SELECTIVITY AND SPECIFICITY

Specificity is the ability to assess unequivocally the analyte in the presence of components, which may be expected to be present. Typically, these might include impurities, degradants, matrix, and so on. Lack of specificity of an individual analytical procedure may be compensated by other supporting analytical procedure(s).

The terms *selectivity* and *specificity* are often used interchangeably. The term *specificity* generally refers to a method that produces a response for single analyte only. Whereas the method, which provides responses for a number of chemical entities that, may or may not be distinguished from each other, is termed as *selective*. If the response is distinguished from all other responses, the method is said to be selective. Since there are very few methods that respond to only one analyte, the term *selectivity* is usually more appropriate.

Selectivity will be achieved in HPLC by choosing optimal columns and setting chromatographic conditions, such as mobile phase composition, column temperature and detector wavelength, and so on.

While performing method validation, at least five potentially interfering substances will be evaluated for potential assay interference. It is worth mentioning that the materials used in the specificity study should be well characterized. When the potentially interfering substances are spiked into the method, recovery should be at least 90% and the relative standard deviation should not exceed 2%.

PRECISION AND REPRODUCIBILITY

The precision of an analytical procedure expresses the closeness of agreement between a series of measurements obtained from multiple sampling of the homogeneous sample under the prescribed conditions. The measured standard deviation can be subdivided into three categories:

a. Repeatability
b. Intermediate precision
c. Reproducibility

Repeatability will be obtained when one operator using one piece of equipment over a relatively short time period carries out the analysis. A minimum of five or six determinations of three different matrixes at two or three different concentrations will be done and the relative standard deviation is calculated. Precision of 1% relative standard deviation (RSD) or less than 1% is easily achievable for compound analysis in pharmaceutical QC. For biological samples the precision is more like 15% at the concentration limits and 10% at other concentration levels.

Intermediate precision expresses within-laboratories variations: different days, different analysts, different equipment, and so on.

Reproducibility represents the precision obtained between laboratories with the objective to verify that the method will provide the same results in different laboratories. The reproducibility of an analytical method will be determined by analysing aliquots from homogeneous lots in different laboratories with different analysts and by using operational and environmental conditions that may differ from but are still within the specified parameters of the method.

Reproducibility could be affected by the following parameters:

1. Different operators with varying level of experience
2. RT and humidity difference

3. Variations in instrument conditions, for example, HPLC model, mobile phase composition and flow rate, pH and so on
4. Different consumables and columns from different suppliers
5. Quality of solvents, reagents and standards

ACCURACY AND RECOVERY

Accuracy of an analytical method is the closeness of agreement between the value, which is accepted either as a conventional true value or as an accepted reference value, and the value found.

The true value for accuracy assessment can be obtained by a comparison of the results of the method with the results from an established reference method. This approach assumes that the uncertainty of the reference method is known. The other way is to spike placebo preparations with varying amounts of active ingredient(s). If a placebo cannot be obtained, then a sample should be spiked at varying levels. After extraction of the analyte from the matrix and injection into the analytical instrument, its recovery will be determined by comparing the response of the extract with the response of the reference material dissolved in a pure solvent. In both cases, acceptable recovery must be demonstrated.

LINEARITY AND CALIBRATION CURVE

The linearity of an analytical procedure is its ability to obtain test results, which are directly proportional to the concentration of analyte in the sample. Linearity test will be performed to give assurance that the method is valid for its intended use throughout the specified ranges.

Linearity of methods will be determined by a series of three to six injections of five or more standards whose concentrations span 80–120% of the expected concentration range. The response should be directly or by means of a well-defined mathematical calculation proportional to the concentrations of the analytes.

Classical linearity acceptance criteria are

1. That the correlation coefficient of the linear regression line is not more than some number close to 1
2. That the y-intercept should not differ significantly from zero

When linear regression analyses are performed, it is important not to force the origin as (0, 0) in the calculation. This practice may significantly skew the actual best-fit slope through the physical range of use.

Frequently the linearity is evaluated graphically in addition or alternatively to mathematical evaluation. The evaluation is made by visual inspection of a plot of signal height or peak area as a function of analyte concentration.

Because deviations from linearity are sometimes difficult to detect, two additional graphical procedures can be used. The first one is to plot the deviations from the regression line versus the concentration or versus the logarithm of the concentration, if the concentration range covers several decades. For linear ranges, the deviations should be equally distributed between positive and negative values.

RANGE

The range of an analytical method is the interval between the upper and lower concentrations of analyte in the sample that have been demonstrated to be determined with precision, accuracy and linearity using the method as written. The range is normally expressed in the same units as the test results (e.g., percentage, parts per million) obtained by the analytical method.

LIMIT OF DETECTION AND QUANTITATION

The quantitation limit of an individual analytical procedure is the lowest amount of analyte in a sample, which can be quantitatively determined with suitable precision and accuracy. The quantitation limit is a parameter of quantitative assays for low levels of compounds in sample matrixes, and is used particularly for the determination of impurities and/or degradation products.

The limit of quantitation is the minimum injected amount that gives precise measurements, in chromatography requiring peak heights 10–20 times higher than baseline noise. A number of samples with decreasing amounts of the analyte will be injected six times. The calculated RSD% of the precision will be plotted against the analyte amount. The amount that corresponds to the previously defined required precision is equal to the limit of quantitation.

ROBUSTNESS

The robustness of an analytical procedure is a measure of its capacity to remain unaffected by small, but deliberate, variations in method parameters and provides an indication of its reliability during normal usage.

For the determination of a method's robustness a number of chromatographic parameters, for example, flow rate, column temperature, injection volume, detection wavelength or mobile phase composition, are varied within a realistic range and the quantitative influence of the variables is determined. If the effect of the parameter is within a specified tolerance, the parameter is said to be within the method's robustness range.

Ideally, robustness is explored during the development of the assay method. By far, the most efficient way to do this is through the use of a designed experiment.

ACCEPTANCE CRITERIA

The determination of limits and acceptance criteria is a crucial element of a good method validation program. A limit as an actual numerical value is one of the requirements of the acceptance criteria of a method validation protocol. Limits and criteria should be

a. Practical
b. Verifiable
c. Achievable
d. Scientifically sound

ANALYTICAL RESULTS REPORTING

The analyst will perform the analysis on the samples as per protocol. The results will be reported to the department manager.

The R&D and QC department managers will give final approval to the reviewed results by signing the final report. Director, QA department will approve the final report.

INCIDENT INVESTIGATION

If there are any validation results that do not meet the acceptance criteria, they are to be investigated through an OOS investigation. If analytical error is excluded as a possible cause of OOS results, then an investigation must be initiated to determine the possible cause of the failure or non-conformance. If necessary, changes should be recommended to prevent a reoccurrence.

VALIDATION REPORTS

Upon completion of the requirements of the analytical method validation protocol, a report will be written summarizing the outcome of the validation. The report will include explanations of any incidents or deviations that may have occurred during the validation study and the actions taken.

A validation report will be prepared that includes:

a. Objective and scope of the method (applicability, type)
b. Type of compounds and matrix
c. Detailed chemicals, reagents, reference standards and control sample preparations
d. Procedures for quality checks of standards and chemicals used
e. Safety considerations
f. Method parameters
g. Critical parameters indicated from robustness testing
h. Listing of equipment and its functional and performance requirements, for example, cell dimensions, baseline noise, and column temperature range

  i. Detailed conditions on how the experiments were conducted, including sample preparation
  j. Statistical procedures and representative calculations
  k. Procedures for QC in the routine (e.g., system suitability tests)
  l. Representative plots, for example, chromatograms, spectra and calibration curves
  m. Method acceptance limit performance data
  n. The expected uncertainty of measurement results
  o. Criteria for revalidation
  p. Person who developed and initially validated the method
  q. Summary and conclusions

CHANGE CONTROL/REVALIDATION

Any changes to the process, analytical method, testing equipment in the SOP QCT-000, or the introduction of a new product, will be documented and its affect on the state of the test method will be determined through change control process. The R&D manager, QC manager and QA manager will review the change and will decide whether revalidation is necessary.

QCT-08
Analytical Methods Validation Protocol

ABC PHARMACEUTICAL COMPANY

Protocol #001

Analytical Method Validation of Assay Technique on HPLC for XYZ Product

Quality Control Department

Primary Author: Analyst

Executed by: Analyst

Approved by: QC Manager

Document Status: Final

Release Date: day/month/year

Number of Pages: 00

PURPOSE

The purpose of this validation protocol is to document that the method for testing various ingredients as outlined in the table below, consistently, reliably and reproducibly provides the expected result.

INTRODUCTION

A new system for qualitative and quantitative assay on HPLC was established for product XYZ that is assayed with different mobile phases. A new method in one system on Gradient HPLC was developed in the QC Department. This method is stable with sharp peaks, good separation and good resolution.

MATERIALS AND EQUIPMENT

CHEMICALS AND REAGENTS

- Purified water, HPLC grade
- Acetonitrile, HPLC grade
- Hexane sulphonic acid sodium salt
- Sodium dihydrogen orthophosphate
- Tetrahydrofuran
- Ortho phosphoric acid

EQUIPMENT

- Analytical balance
- Volumetric glassware, Class A
- pH meter
- Sonicator
- Vacuum pump and filtration assembly for mobile phase

CHROMATOGRAPHIC CONDITIONS

- System: Perkin Elmer, Gradient HPLC system equipped with a variable UV–Visible detector, an autoinjector, and total chrome software.
- Column: C-18, 250 × 4.6 mm, 5-μm (SGE C18) or equivalent.
- Mobile phase.
  Buffer: About 4 g of sodium dihydrogen phosphate salt and 0.5 g of hexane sulphonic acid sodium were taken in a 1000-ml volumetric flask; about 900 mL of distilled water was added. It was shaken and pH was adjusted to 3.0 with diluted phosphoric acid.
  Mobile phase (A): (BUFFER: ACETONITRILE: THF) (900:40:4) V/V
  Mobile phase (B): (BUFFER: ACETONITRILE: THF) (600:400:3) V/V
  Filtered through 0.45 μm membrane filter and

GRADIENT COMPOSITION OF MOBILE PHASE

Step Time	Time	Flow Rate	Mobile Phase A	Mobile Phase B	Curve	Wavelength (nm)
0						
1						
2						
3						
4						

- Post run time: X min
- Injection vol.: X-μL
- Detection: UV, XX nm
- Temperature: Ambient
- Diluents: Water

RESPONSIBILITIES

QC analysts will perform the tests according to the approved protocol.

The protocol will be reviewed by QC assistant manager and approved by QC manager and QA director.

All the tests will be performed in the QC laboratory.

DEFINITIONS

Specificity: The ability to assess the analyte in the presence of components that may be expected to be present, for example, impurities, degradants, and so on, is called specificity of the method.

Accuracy: This term expresses the closeness of agreement between the accepted reference value and the value found.

Precision: The closeness of agreement between a series of measurements obtained from sampling of the same homogeneous sample under the prescribed conditions.

Repeatability: This term expresses the precision under the same operating conditions over a short interval of time.

Detection limit: It is the lowest amount of analyte in a sample that can be detected but not necessarily quantitated as an exact value.

Quantitation limit: The lowest amount of analyte in a sample that can be quantitatively determined with suitable precision and accuracy.

Linearity: Assay's ability (within a given range) to obtain test results that are directly proportional to the concentration (amount) of analyte in the sample.

Robustness: It is a measure of the assay capacity to remain unaffected by small but deliberate variations in method parameters and provides an indication of its reliability during normal usage.

PROCEDURE

1. **Calibration curve:** Will be determined by a series of five injections of five or more standards whose concentration span is 80–120% of the expected concentration range.

   Acceptance criteria: A linear regression equation applied to the results should have an intercept not significantly different from zero.

2. **Precision:** System suitability or precision is an integral part of many analytical procedures. The precision of this method will be determined by analysing five test samples prepared as directed in the test preparations. This test will be performed by carrying out the analysis by
   - Two different analysts
   - Over a period of 1 week
   - Using two different columns
   - Two different machines

   Acceptance criteria: The relative standard deviation of assay results should not be more than 2%.

3. **Accuracy (recovery):** The accuracy or recovery of the method will be determined by spiking different levels of target concentration of the active ingredients, under study, standard solution to the placebo mixture of the respective products. This mixture will then be treated as test solution by the HPLC method. The accuracy of the method over 50–150% of target concentration will be measured by calculating the recovery of each ingredient by the following equation:

$$\text{Percentage of recovery} = \frac{\text{Amount of ingredient found}}{\text{Amount of ingredient added}} \times 100$$

   Acceptance criteria: The percent of recovery should be within 95–105%.

4. **Linearity and ranges:** The linearity test will be performed to give assurance that the method is valid for its intended use throughout the specified ranges. Incremental concentration of standard solution containing the active ingredients of the specific product will be prepared in the working range that is, about 25–200% of the analysing concentration (target concentration) to verify that the response is proportionately linear.

   Standard solution of different strengths will be prepared and run on HPLC. Corresponding peak areas of the active ingredients will be recorded and plotting response against concentration will draw calibration graphs.

5. **Robustness:** Robustness tests will be performed to examine the effect that operational parameters have on the analysis results.

   For the determination of method robustness, a number of chromatographic parameters, for example, flow rate, injection volume and detection wavelength will be varied within a realistic range and the quantitative influence of variables will be determined. All these variables will be described in detail in the validation report.

Acceptance criteria: The influence of the parameter should be within the method's robustness range.

Final report: A final report will be written after the successful completion of all the tests discussed in this protocol. The final report will include an executive summary and a results and discussion section which will encompass all the tests, their results and inference made from the results. A final conclusion will also be made in regard to the method successfully validated and recommended for intended use.

The final report will be reviewed and approved by QC manager and QA director as a minimum.

QCT-09

SOP for Annual Re-Qualification of HPLC Units

PURPOSE

The purpose of this SOP is to provide written instructions to perform annual re-qualification of HPLC units in QC Department at ABC Pharmaceutical Company.

SCOPE

The scope of this SOP applies to all new and existing HPLC units used in the analyses of finished products and raw materials in QC Laboratory.

RESPONSIBILITIES

The QC assistant manager/designate is responsible to perform re-qualification, whereas the QC manager will be responsible for the compliance of this SOP.

HPLC QUALIFICATION

The GMP requires the precision and accuracy of analytical instruments to obtain valid data for research, development, manufacturing and QC. The regulations also require the companies to establish procedures assuring that the instruments that generate data supporting regulated product testing are fit for use.

Following the initial qualification, the annual re-qualification of the HPLC units will be performed in house. All HPLC units will be re-qualified every year. The frequency of performing re-qualification will be 1 year ± 2 months. Once the re-qualification is completed, a report will be compiled and will be reviewed by the QC manager/designate (as appropriate) as well as by the QA manager/designate and will be approved by the QA director as a minimum.

ABC PHARMACEUTICAL COMPANY

STANDARD OPERATING PROCEDURE

	SOP No.: ABC-000
Subject: SOP for Annual Re-Qualification of HPLC Units in Quality Control Department	Revision No.: 0

ATTACHMENT

Form No. 1

PROCEDURE

An HPLC unit comprises of the following parts:

1. Auto sampler
2. Pump
3. Detector

In order to perform re-qualification, tests for the different parts of HPLC will be performed in the following way:

TESTS FOR AN AUTO SAMPLER

Linearity (for UV & Diode Array Spectrophotometer)

To test the linearity of the auto sampler, the process will be performed as follows:
  a. Adjust the following with the HPLC system
    i.   Mobile phase—70% acetonitrile in water
    ii. Column—μ Bondapack C_{18}, 10 μm
    iii. Wavelength—275 nm
    iv. Flow rate—1 mL/min
    v.   Injection volume—20 μL
  b. Standard preparation
    i. Dissolve 10 mg caffeine in water in a 100-mL volumetric flask.
    ii. Dilute 1 mL of the above solution with water in a 100-mL volumetric flask (Concentration 1 mg%, Solution A).
  c. Procedure
    i. Inject multiple injection volume (10, 20, 30, 40 and 50 μL) from the same sample; R-square should be greater than or equal to 0.999.

Repeatability (Precision) (for UV and Diode Array Spectrophotometers)

Follow the steps as shown below to perform the repeatability test:
  a. Using the same HPLC system in the linearity test, inject (Solution A) 10 times. The % RSD should be below 1%.

ABC PHARMACEUTICAL COMPANY

STANDARD OPERATING PROCEDURE

	SOP No.: ABC-000
Subject: SOP for Annual Re-Qualification of HPLC Units in Quality Control Department	Revision No.: 0

Carry-over (for UV and Diode Array Spectrophotometer)

Carry-over is the amount of the previous sample retained by the system in the current sample. The specification of this test is less than or equal to 0.02%

$$\text{To calculate carry-over: } \frac{\text{Area of blank}}{\text{Area of sample}} \times 100$$

TESTS FOR PUMP

Flow Accuracy Test (for UV and Diode Array Spectrophotometer)

The flow accuracy test is used to prove that the flow rate selected on the pump is delivered in the correct time.

    a. Disconnect the column and run the pump with 70% acetonitrile.

    b. Check the flow rate of pump A, pump B and the gradient system as 50% pump A and 50% pump B using a flow rate of 1.0 mL/min.

    c. Measure the time required for a 10-mL cylinder.

    d. Calculate the actual flow rate as follows:

$$\text{Actual flow rate : } \frac{10}{T \text{ (time)}}$$

$$\text{Acceptance criteria} = 1 \pm 0.05 \text{ mL/min } (\pm 5\%)$$

Composition Accuracy Test (for UV and Diode Array Spectrophotometer)

The composition accuracy test proves that the proportioning valves are operating correctly.

    Adjust the HPLC system as follows:

        a. Disconnect the column (put connection between the pump and the detector).

ABC PHARMACEUTICAL COMPANY

STANDARD OPERATING PROCEDURE

	SOP No.: ABC-000
Subject: SOP for Annual Re-Qualification of HPLC Units in Quality Control Department	Revision No.: 0

   b. Prepare a solution of 0.2% acetone in water (Note: for the diode array detector, prepare 0.1% acetone solution).
   c. Fill reservoir A with water.
   d. Fill reservoir B with acetone solution.
   e. Wavelength: 265 nm.
   f. Pump the acetone solution through reservoir B for 30 min at a flow rate of 5 mL/min.
   g. Generate and run the method in the table, record detector absorbance values for each step (Auto zero the detector after Step 1).

Step	Time (min)	Flow (mL/min)	%A	%B	Curve	AU
0	5.0	5.0	100	0	0	
1	1.0	5.0	100	0	0	
2	3.0	5.0	0	100	0	AU1
3	3.0	5.0	10	90	0	AU2
4	3.0	5.0	49	51	0	AU3
5	3.0	5.0	51	49	0	AU4
6	3.0	5.0	90	10	0	AU5

Calculate the composition (C):

$$C(90) = \frac{AU2}{AU1} \times 100$$

$$C(51) = \frac{AU3}{AU1} \times 100$$

$$C(49) = \frac{AU4}{AU1} \times 100$$

$$C(10) = \frac{AU5}{AU1} \times 100$$

Record the composition accuracy (C) for every step; the limit should be within ±1.0% of the target %.

ABC PHARMACEUTICAL COMPANY

STANDARD OPERATING PROCEDURE

	SOP No.: ABC-000
Subject: SOP for Annual Re-Qualification of HPLC Units in Quality Control Department	Revision No.: 0

TESTS FOR DETECTOR

Wavelength Accuracy (for UV Spectrophotometer)

To perform the Wavelength Accuracy test, adjust the HPLC system in the following way:

a. Disconnect the column (put any connector between the pump and the detector).
b. Prepare the following solution (10 mg caffeine in 1000 mL water), that is, 1 mg%.
c. Fill reservoir A with water.
d. Fill reservoir B with caffeine solution.
e. Flow rate: 3 mL/min.
f. Injection volume: 10 µL (from caffeine solution).
g. Make the following pump parameters:

Step	Time (min)	Flow (mL/min)	%A	%B	Curve
0	5.0	3.0	100	0	0
1	1.0	3.0	100	0	0
2	23	3.0	0	100	0

h. Make the following detector parameters:

Step	Time (min)	Wavelength (nm)	Auto Zero	Step	Time (min)	Wavelength (nm)	Auto Zero
1	1.0	300	No	11	1.0	269	No
2	4.0	200	No	12	1.0	270	No
3	1.0	201	No	13	1.0	271	No
4	1.0	202	No	14	1.0	272	No
5	1.0	203	No	15	1.0	273	No
6	1.0	204	No	16	1.0	274	No
7	1.0	205	No	17	1.0	275	No
8	1.0	206	No	18	1.0	276	No
9	1.0	207	No	19	1.0	277	No
10	1.0	208	No	20	1.0	278	No

ABC PHARMACEUTICAL COMPANY

STANDARD OPERATING PROCEDURE

	SOP No.: ABC-000
Subject: SOP for Annual Re-Qualification of HPLC Units in Quality Control Department	Revision No.: 0

The maximum wavelength peaks for caffeine should be at 205 and 273 nm.

   i. The acceptance criteria for wavelengths 205 ± 1 and 273 ± 1 nm

Wavelength Accuracy (for Diode Array Spectrophotometer)

Adjust the following HPLC system:

   a. Column: μ Bonda pack C18 10 μm.
   b. Mobile phase: 70% acetonitrile.
   c. Flow rate: 1 mL/min.
   d. Wavelength range: 200–400 nm.
   e. Injection volume: 20 μL.
   f. Inject caffeine solution 1 mg% (solution A).
   g. The caffeine shows two maxima at wavelengths 205 and 273 nm.
   h. The acceptance criteria is 205 ± 2 and 273 ± 2 nm.

ABC PHARMACEUTICAL COMPANY

STANDARD OPERATING PROCEDURE

Subject: SOP for Annual Re-Qualification of HPLC Units in Quality Control Department	SOP No.: ABC-000
	Revision No.: 0

FORM NO. 1

HPLC QUALIFICATION CERTIFICATE

I. Auto Sample

1. Linearity

Result (R-square:) (Limit ≥ 0.999)

2. Repeatability

Result (%RSD:.............) (Limit < 1%)

3. Carry-Over

Result (............) (Limit ≤ 0.02%)

II. Pump

1. Flow Accuracy Test

Result (............) (Limit 1 ± 0.05 mL/min)

2. Composition Accuracy Test

I $\dfrac{AU2}{AU1} \times 100 =$ .... (Limit 90% ± 1%)

II $\dfrac{AU3}{AU1} \times 100 =$ .... (Limit 51% ± 1%)

III $\dfrac{AU4}{AU1} \times 100 =$ .... (Limit 49% ± 1%)

IV $\dfrac{AU5}{AU1} \times 100 =$ .... (Limit 10% ± 1%)

ABC PHARMACEUTICAL COMPANY

STANDARD OPERATING PROCEDURE

	SOP No.: ABC-000
Subject: SOP for Annual Re-Qualification of HPLC Units in Quality Control Department	Revision No.: 0

III. Detector

1. Wavelength Accuracy for UV Spectrophotometers

Result at 205 nm: --------------- (Limit 205 ± 1 nm)

Result at 273 nm: --------------- (Limit 273 ± 1 nm)

2. Wavelength Accuracy for Diode Array Spectrophotometers

Result at 205 nm: --------------- (Limit 205 ± 2 nm)

Result at 273 nm: --------------- (Limit 273 ± 2 nm)

QCT-10
SOP for Annual Re-Qualification of GC Units

PURPOSE

The purpose of this SOP is to provide written instructions to perform annual re-qualification of GC units in QC, R&D and stability study departments.

SCOPE

The scope of this SOP applies to all new and existing GC units used in the analysis of finished product and raw materials in the laboratories of ABC Pharmaceutical Company.

RESPONSIBILITIES

QC assistant managers/designates are responsible to perform re-qualification, whereas the laboratory manager will be responsible for the compliance of this SOP.

HPLC QUALIFICATION

The GMP requires the precision and accuracy of analytical instruments to obtain valid data for R&D, manufacturing and QC. The regulations also require the companies to establish procedures assuring that the instruments that generate data supporting regulated product testing are fit for use.

Following the initial qualification, the annual re-qualification of the GC units will be performed in-house. All GC units will be re-qualified every year. The frequency of performing re-qualification will be 1 year ± 2 months. Once the re-qualification is completed, a report will be compiled and will be reviewed by the QC manager/designate (as appropriate) as well as by QA manager/designate and will be approved by the QA director as a minimum.

ABC PHARMACEUTICAL COMPANY

STANDARD OPERATING PROCEDURE

	SOP No.: ABC-000
Subject: SOP for Annual Re-Qualification of GC Units in Quality Control Department	Revision No.: 0

ATTACHMENT

Form No. 1

PROCEDURE

A GC unit comprises of the following parts:

1. Auto sampler
2. Pump
3. Detector

In order to perform re-qualification, tests for the different parts of HPLC will be performed in the following way:

1. FLOW RATE VERIFICATION TEST

a. Install an appropriate test column into the injector and the detector.
b. Set the carrier pneumatic flow to the value.
c. By using a calibrated flow meter measure the flow of the column.
d. Cap off the detector and record the flow.
e. If the difference in readings is more than ±20% of set flow, adjustment is required.

2. TEMPERATURE VERIFICATION TEST

a. Enter injector/detector set temperature points (e.g., 150°C).
b. Insert a calibrated temperature probe into the oven near the oven sensor.
c. Allow all zones to stabilize and the instrument to become ready.
d. Record the actual temperature probe value and the displayed values for the injector/detector zones of the oven temperature.
e. If the difference is more than ±0.5°C, adjustment is required.

ABC PHARMACEUTICAL COMPANY

STANDARD OPERATING PROCEDURE

Subject: SOP for Annual Re-Qualification of GC Units in Quality Control Department	SOP No.: ABC-000
	Revision No.: 0

3. DETECTOR EVALUATION TEST

a. Stabilize the system first by making multiple runs, and then select one of these runs to perform the detector sensitivity evaluation.

b. Prepare one vial of test mix; manually inject 0.5 µL of the test mix.

c. Calculate the sensitivity S in Coulombs/gram. It should be more than ≥ 0.01 C/g. If not, adjustment should be done, and the test must be repeated.

Attachment –1

Instrument	Model No.	Serial No.	Location

1-Flow Rate Verification Test

Parameter	Set Flow	Monitor Flow Before Adjustment	Monitor Flow After Adjustment	Difference	Acceptance Criteria	Result (Pass/Fail)
					± 20%	

2-Temperature Verification Test

Parameter	Set Temperature	Monitor Temperature Before Adjustment	Monitor Temperature After Adjustment	Difference	Acceptance Criteria	Result (Pass/Fail)
Detector					± 0.5°C	
Injector					± 0.5°C	

3-Detector Evaluation Test

Detector	Detector Sensitivity Spec.	Detector Final Result	Result (Pass/Fail)
	≥ 0.01 C/g		

Done by: **Verified by:**

ABC PHARMACEUTICAL COMPANY

STANDARD OPERATING PROCEDURE

	SOP No.: ABC-000
Subject: SOP for Annual Re-Qualification of GC Units in Quality Control Department	Revision No.: 0

Repeatability (Precision) (for UV and Diode Array Spectrophotometers)

Follow the steps as shown below to perform the repeatability test:

   a. Using the same HPLC system in the linearity test, inject (solution A) 10 times. The % RSD should be below 1%.

Carry-Over (for UV and Diode Array Spectrophotometer)

Carry-over is the amount of the previous sample retained by the system in the current sample. The specification of this test is less than or equal to 0.02%

$$\text{To calculate carry-over: } \frac{\text{Area of blank}}{\text{Area of sample}} \times 100$$

TESTS FOR PUMP

Flow Accuracy Test (for UV and Diode Array Spectrophotometer)

The flow accuracy test is used to prove that the flow rate selected on the pump is delivered in the correct time.

   a. Disconnect the column and run the pump with 70% acetonitrile.
   b. Check the flow rate of pump A, pump B and the gradient system as 50% pump A and 50% pump B using a flow rate of 1.0 mL/min.
   c. Measure the time required for a 10-mL cylinder.
   d. Calculate the actual flow rate as follows:

$$\text{Actual flow rate: } \frac{10}{T \ (\text{time})}$$

Acceptance criteria = 1 ± 0.05 mL/min ($\pm 5\%$)

Composition Accuracy Test (for UV and Diode Array Spectrophotometer)

The composition accuracy test proves that the proportioning valves are operating correctly.

ABC PHARMACEUTICAL COMPANY

STANDARD OPERATING PROCEDURE

Subject: SOP for Annual Re-Qualification of GC Units in Quality Control Department	SOP No.: ABC-000
	Revision No.: 0

Adjust the HPLC system as follows:

a. Disconnect the column (put connection between the pump and the detector).
b. Prepare a solution of 0.2% acetone in water (Note: for the diode array detector, prepare 0.1% acetone solution).
c. Fill reservoir A with water.
d. Fill reservoir B with acetone solution.
e. Wavelength: 265 nm.
f. Pump the acetone solution through reservoir B for 30 min at a flow rate of 5 mL/min.
g. Generate and run the method in the table, record detector absorbance values for each step (Auto zero the detector after Step 1).

Step	Time (min)	Flow (mL/min)	%A	%B	Curve	AU
0	5.0	5.0	100	0	0	
1	1.0	5.0	100	0	0	
2	3.0	5.0	0	100	0	AU1
3	3.0	5.0	10	90	0	AU2
4	3.0	5.0	49	51	0	AU3
5	3.0	5.0	51	49	0	AU4
6	3.0	5.0	90	10	0	AU5

Calculate the composition (C):

$$C(90) = \frac{AU2}{AU1} \times 100$$

$$C(51) = \frac{AU3}{AU1} \times 100$$

$$C(49) = \frac{AU4}{AU1} \times 100$$

$$C(10) = \frac{AU5}{AU1} \times 100$$

ABC PHARMACEUTICAL COMPANY

STANDARD OPERATING PROCEDURE

	SOP No.: ABC-000
Subject: SOP for Annual Re-Qualification of GC Units in Quality Control Department	Revision No.: 0

Record the composition accuracy (C) for every step; the limit should be within ±1.0% of the target %.

TESTS FOR DETECTOR

Wavelength Accuracy (for UV Spectrophotometer)

To perform the wavelength accuracy test, adjust the HPLC system in the following way:

a. Disconnect the column (put any connector between the pump and the detector).

b. Prepare the following solution (10 mg caffeine in 1000 mL water)—that is, 1 mg%.

c. Fill reservoir A with water.

d. Fill reservoir B with caffeine solution.

e. Flow rate: 3 mL/min.

f. Injection volume: 10 μL (from caffeine solution).

g. Make the following pump parameters.

Step	Time (min)	Flow (mL/min)	%A	%B	Curve
0	5.0	3.0	100	0	0
1	1.0	3.0	100	0	0
2	23	3.0	0	100	0

a. Make the following detector parameters:

Step	Time (min)	Wavelength (nm)	Auto Zero	Step	Time (min)	Wavelength (nm)	Auto Zero
1	1.0	300	No	11	1.0	269	No
2	4.0	200	No	12	1.0	270	No
3	1.0	201	No	13	1.0	271	No
4	1.0	202	No	14	1.0	272	No
5	1.0	203	No	15	1.0	273	No

ABC PHARMACEUTICAL COMPANY

STANDARD OPERATING PROCEDURE

	SOP No.: ABC-000
Subject: SOP for Annual Re-Qualification of GC Units in Quality Control Department	Revision No.: 0

6	1.0	204	No	16	1.0	274	No
7	1.0	205	No	17	1.0	275	No
8	1.0	206	No	18	1.0	276	No
9	1.0	207	No	19	1.0	277	No
10	1.0	208	No	20	1.0	278	No

b. The maximum wavelength peaks for caffeine should be at 205 and 273 nm.
c. The acceptance criteria for wavelengths 205 ± 1 and 273 ± 1 nm.

Wavelength Accuracy (for Diode Array Spectrophotometer)
Adjust the following HPLC system:

a. Column: μ Bonda pack C18 10 μm.
b. Mobile phase: 70% acetonitrile.
c. Flow rate: 1 mL/min.
d. Wavelength range: 200–400 nm.
e. Injection volume: 20 μL.
f. Inject caffeine solution 1 mg% (solution A).
g. The caffeine shows two maxima at wavelengths 205 and 273 nm.
h. The acceptance criteria is 205 ± 2 and 273 ± 2 nm.

FORM NO. 1

HPLC Qualification Certificate

  I. Auto Sample
    1. Linearity

             Result (*R*-square): (Limit ≥ 0.999)
    2. Repeatability

             Result (%RSD): (Limit <1%)
    3. Carry-over

             Result (.................................) (Limit ≤ 0.02%)

ABC PHARMACEUTICAL COMPANY

STANDARD OPERATING PROCEDURE

	SOP No.: ABC-000
Subject: SOP for Annual Re-Qualification of GC Units in Quality Control Department	Revision No.: 0

II. Pump

1. Flow Accuracy Test

Result (.............................) (Limit 1 ± 0.05 mL/min)

2. Composition Accuracy Test

I $\dfrac{AU2}{AU1} \times 100 = \ldots\ldots\ldots\ldots\ldots$ (Limit 90% ± 1%)

II $\dfrac{AU3}{AU1} \times 100 = \ldots\ldots\ldots\ldots\ldots$ (Limit 51% ± 1%)

III $\dfrac{AU4}{AU1} \times 100 = \ldots\ldots\ldots\ldots\ldots$ (Limit 49% ± 1%)

IV $\dfrac{AU5}{AU1} \times 100 = \ldots\ldots\ldots\ldots\ldots$ (Limit 10% ± 1%)

III. Detector

1. Wavelength Accuracy for UV Spectrophotometers

Result at 205 nm: ----------------(Limit 205 ±1 nm)

Result at 273 nm: ----------------(Limit 273 ±1 nm)

2. Wavelength Accuracy for Diode Array Spectrophotometers

Result at 205 nm: ----------------(Limit 205 ± 2 nm)

Result at 273 nm: ----------------(Limit 273 ± 2 nm)

Done by: _____

Approved by: _____

Quality Control Manager

QCT-11
ABC Pharmaceutical Company

GOOD LABORATORY PRACTICES

The following is a checklist of GLPs in the QC laboratory to be followed as guidelines. All employees working in the lab are responsible to follow the procedure. All assistants and deputy managers as well as section supervisors are responsible for implementing the procedure.

GENERAL

Check the following:

1. The chemists/analysts are medically examined and cleared before being allowed to work in the area.
2. Analysts in the area wear protective lab coats, clogs and safety goggles.
3. The designated person keeps all working areas clean as per the respective SOPs.
4. No eating, smoking or unhygienic practices are allowed in the laboratory.
5. Keep the lockers provided in the facility clean. Do not keep unwanted items inside the lockers, only prescribed medicines are allowed. Keep street shoes and personal clothes segregated from the laboratory clogs and gowns.
6. All apparatuses and equipment used in the laboratory are cleaned and calibrated as per the specific SOPs. Each of the equipment has a status label.
7. Clearly legible labels having all the required information identify the contents of all containers used in the laboratory during the analytical work.
8. All respective SOPs are current and followed. Each analyst is responsible for his SOPs reading records once per year or after any change is made.
9. Primary and secondary reference standards, chemical and reagents issue records are maintained.

10. Volumetric solutions preparation records are maintained.
11. All the laboratory rooms have required temperature, relative humidity (Rh) and air pressures to ensure that the work place is comfortable and appropriate for test samples.
12. Weighing and measuring of materials is done on balances with printers and all the printouts are available with the analyst's working registers.
13. All incoming samples of raw material, packaging commodities, bulk and finished products are stored as per SOPs in the respective area until issued for analysis.
14. Weekly and monthly register checking is done.
15. Assistant managers must inspect glass apparatus on a weekly basis and section supervisors must ensure that all broken glassware have been discarded.
16. Cleaning of the area is done according to schedule and specific SOPs and is documented.
17. File sample room's temperature and Rh records must be checked and reviewed on a monthly basis.
18. Destruction of expired file samples and the records reviewed should be done on a monthly basis.
19. Maintenance of records and usage of logbooks for each HPLC column, available in the QC inventory are appropriately checked on a regular basis.
20. Logbooks and daily calibration records of weighing balances are updated daily after performing the calibration.
21. Storage of the raw materials, packaging materials, bulk products and finished products is as per the specific SOPs with proper temperature monitoring and recording.
22. All revalidation records of autoclaves are checked every month.
23. All refrigerator temperature records are monitored, reviewed and checked on a regular basis.
24. Media preparation and destruction records are maintained and checked regularly.
25. Personal hygiene records/excursion records are maintained for all manufacturing areas on a monthly basis.
26. All autoclaves revalidation records are maintained.
27. Growth promotion tests are being carried out for every prepared lot of growth media.
28. Solvents disposal records are maintained on a monthly basis.
29. All the logbooks are updated.
30. Temperature indicators have valid calibration tags.
31. All vessels and utensils are labelled as to their cleanliness status.
32. STMs are at hand during analysis, and are updated, approved and accurately followed.
33. All products are tested as per approved specifications and STMs being adhered to.

34. Mobile phase vessels should be labelled with the name and date of preparation and expiry on them.
35. Analysts should report the OOS results immediately to their supervisors who in turn should prompt investigation and inform the manager or director.
36. Any probable delay in testing by more than one day should be immediately brought to notice of the manager.
37. DI water and WFI chemical analysis trend report/month and microbiological analysis with excursions published and recorded are maintained on a regular basis.
38. Utilities lines in the laboratory (where available) are clearly marked and labelled.
39. All records must be completed at the time of action.
40. Employees have full knowledge about their job functions.
41. The department is well maintained and is spacious enough for equipment and other analytical work.
42. Area and equipment are cleaned at the end of the day.
43. Specific procedures for cleaning of major equipments are followed.

GOOD DOCUMENTATION SKILLS

1. The correct ink colour and type and proper writing instrument are used (pencils should not be used).
2. Additional documents (e.g., charts, printouts) are properly included with batch number, product name, signature and date.
3. The printing and writing can be easily read.
4. Errors are properly corrected with one line through the original entry, initiated, dated and explained (if necessary).
5. Calculations are reviewed and verified.
6. Numbers are properly rounded off; the correct significant figures are used.
7. All measurable results must be entered in the Certificate of Analysis instead of merely "Conform" or "Passes" statements.
8. Spelling of the product names and other words are correct.
9. Proper formats for date and time are used (date/month/year).
10. All abbreviations are approved and standardized.
11. Blank spaces are properly handled by putting not applicable (N/A); dash ("—").
12. Each column in the analyst's register is filled in correctly or N/A and must not be left blank.
13. Good documentation skill should produce proper records with the following characteristics:
    a. Permanent
    b. Accurate
    c. Prompt

    d. Clear
    e. Consistent
    f. Complete
    g. Direct
    h. Truthful

GOOD LABORATORY PRACTICES IN MICROBIOLOGY LABORATORY

1. Employees working in sterile testing areas should be appropriately clothed according to the relevant SOPs.
2. Sterile testing areas should be in good shape and neat.
3. Relevant cleaning procedures for area and equipment should be followed.
4. Cleaning and sanitization agents as per the SOP should be labelled with the expiration date.
5. Records are maintained for the preparation of cleaning and sanitization agents.
6. Products and product components must not be exposed unless protected under Laminar Flow Hood Air.
7. Handling and other working practices should be devoid of contamination and generation of particles.
8. All vessels and utensils are labelled appropriately.
9. Microbiological test methods that are at hand during testing are approved and followed accurately.
10. Vessels should be labelled with the product lot number and other information as appropriate.
11. Relevant sterilization and other charts and printouts must be fully labelled, verified and approved.
12. Valid calibration labels should be pasted on all equipment.
13. Material holding containers are intact and can be closed completely.
14. Temperature and humidity are under controlled limits.
15. Utility lines are clearly marked and labelled.
16. Storage of samples (raw, bulk and finished) is maintained under labelled or prescribed storage conditions.
17. All records must be completed at the time of action.
18. All reports are dated correctly and duly signed without delay.

    a. Dos and don'ts to be followed:
      1. Do wear the identification card all the time at work.
      2. Follow safety instructions before entering the lab.
      3. Do read, understand and follow SOPs related to your work.
      4. Do observe personal hygiene at work.
      5. Do keep your nails clean and tidy every week.
      6. Do get your hair cut every month.
      7. Do keep your beard trimmed every day before coming to work.

b. Things that shall not be practiced are described as follows
1. Do not take food and drinks inside the laboratory; specially do not chew gum.
2. Do not enter the laboratory in street shoes and without lab coats.
3. Do not use any unwritten procedure for analysis and follow the basic principle of "Do as it is written and write what you do" and "If it is not written, it was never done."
4. Do not enter into the plant, if suffering from some contagious disease or a lesion over the skin.
5. Do not hold anti-dust facemask, disposable hand gloves and other working tools in your lockers.
6. Do not store medicines inside the locker, except prescribed for personal use by the doctor.
7. Do not carry batch record and support documents in your pockets and lockers.

I have read the memorandum to avoid mistakes during analytical work. I take complete responsibility especially in the event of any deviation from the given instructions leading to non-compliance.

Name & Signature:_____   **Designation:**_____

ID No.: _____   **Department:**_____

Date:_____

QCT-12
Regulations

QCT-12.1

TITLE 21—FOOD AND DRUGS

CHAPTER I—FOOD AND DRUG ADMINISTRATION

DEPARTMENT OF HEALTH AND HUMAN SERVICES

SUBCHAPTER C—DRUGS: GENERAL

PART 211 CURRENT GOOD MANUFACTURING PRACTICE FOR
FINISHED PHARMACEUTICALS

SUBPART I—LABORATORY CONTROLS

Sec. 211.160. General requirements

a. The establishment of any specifications, standards, sampling plans, test
procedures, or other laboratory control mechanisms required by this subpart, including any change in such specifications, standards, sampling
plans, test procedures, or other laboratory control mechanisms, shall be
drafted by the appropriate organizational unit and reviewed and approved
by the quality control unit. The requirements in this subpart shall be followed and shall be documented at the time of performance. Any deviation
from the written specifications, standards, sampling plans, test procedures
or other laboratory control mechanisms shall be recorded and justified.

b. Laboratory controls shall include the establishment of scientifically sound
and appropriate specifications, standards, sampling plans, and test procedures designed to assure that components, drug product containers,
closures, in-process materials, labelling and drug products conform to
appropriate standards of identity, strength, quality and purity. Laboratory
controls shall include:

1. Determination of conformity to applicable written specifications for
the acceptance of each lot within each shipment of components, drug
product containers, closures and labelling used in the manufacture,
processing, packing or holding of drug products. The specifications
shall include a description of the sampling and testing procedures
used. Samples shall be representative and adequately identified. Such

procedures shall also require appropriate retesting of any component, drug product container, or closure that is subject to deterioration.

2. Determination of conformance to written specifications and a description of sampling and testing procedures for in-process materials. Such samples shall be representative and properly identified.

3. Determination of conformance to written descriptions of sampling procedures and appropriate specifications for drug products. Such samples shall be representative and properly identified.

4. The calibration of instruments, apparatus, gauges, and recording devices at suitable intervals in accordance with an established written program containing specific directions, schedules, limits for accuracy and precision, and provisions for remedial action in the event accuracy and/or precision limits are not met. Instruments, apparatus, gauges and recording devices not meeting established specifications shall not be used.

[43 FR 45077, Sept. 29, 1978, as amended at 73 FR 51932, Sept. 8, 2008]

Sec. 211.165. Testing and release for distribution

a. For each batch of drug product, there shall be appropriate laboratory determination of satisfactory conformance to final specifications for the drug product, including the identity and strength of each active ingredient, prior to release. Where sterility and/or pyrogen testing are conducted on specific batches of shortlived radiopharmaceuticals, such batches may be released prior to completion of sterility and/or pyrogen testing, provided such testing is completed as soon as possible.

b. There shall be appropriate laboratory testing, as necessary, of each batch of drug product required to be free of objectionable microorganisms.

c. Any sampling and testing plans shall be described in written procedures that shall include the method of sampling and the number of units per batch to be tested; such written procedure shall be followed.

d. Acceptance criteria for the sampling and testing conducted by the quality control unit shall be adequate to assure that batches of drug products meet each appropriate specification and appropriate statistical quality control criteria as a condition for their approval and release. The statistical quality control criteria shall include appropriate acceptance levels and/or appropriate rejection levels.

e. The accuracy, sensitivity, specificity and reproducibility of test methods employed by the firm shall be established and documented. Such validation and documentation may be accomplished in accordance with 211.194(a)(2).

f. Drug products failing to meet established standards or specifications and any other relevant quality control criteria shall be rejected. Reprocessing may be performed. Prior to acceptance and use, reprocessed material must meet appropriate standards, specifications and any other relevant critieria.

Sec. 211.166. Stability testing

a. There shall be a written testing program designed to assess the stability characteristics of drug products. The results of such stability testing shall be used in determining appropriate storage conditions and expiration dates. The written program shall be followed and shall include:
   1. Sample size and test intervals based on statistical criteria for each attribute examined to assure valid estimates of stability;
   2. Storage conditions for samples retained for testing;
   3. Reliable, meaningful and specific test methods;
   4. Testing of the drug product in the same container-closure system as that in which the drug product is marketed;
   5. Testing of drug products for reconstitution at the time of dispensing (as directed in the labelling) as well as after they are reconstituted.

b. An adequate number of batches of each drug product shall be tested to determine an appropriate expiration date and a record of such data shall be maintained. Accelerated studies, combined with basic stability information on the components, drug products and container-closure system, may be used to support tentative expiration dates provided full shelf life studies are not available and are being conducted. Where data from accelerated studies are used to project a tentative expiration date that is beyond a date supported by actual shelf life studies, there must be stability studies conducted, including drug product testing at appropriate intervals, until the tentative expiration date is verified or the appropriate expiration date determined.

c. For homeopathic drug products, the requirements of this section are as follows:
   1. There shall be a written assessment of stability based at least on testing or examination of the drug product for compatibility of the ingredients, and based on marketing experience with the drug product to indicate that there is no degradation of the product for the normal or expected period of use.
   2. Evaluation of stability shall be based on the same container-closure system in which the drug product is being marketed.

d. Allergenic extracts that are labelled "No U.S. Standard of Potency" are exempt from the requirements of this section.

[43 FR 45077, Sept. 29, 1978, as amended at 46 FR 56412, Nov. 17, 1981]

Sec. 211.167. Special testing requirements

a. For each batch of drug product purporting to be sterile and/or pyrogen-free, there shall be appropriate laboratory testing to determine conformance to such requirements. The test procedures shall be in writing and shall be followed.

b. For each batch of ophthalmic ointment, there shall be appropriate testing to determine conformance to specifications regarding the presence of foreign particles and harsh or abrasive substances. The test procedures shall be in writing and shall be followed.

c. For each batch of controlled-release dosage form, there shall be appropriate laboratory testing to determine conformance to the specifications for the rate of release of each active ingredient. The test procedures shall be in writing and shall be followed.

Sec. 211.170. Reserve samples

a. An appropriately identified reserve sample that is representative of each lot in each shipment of each active ingredient shall be retained. The reserve sample consists of at least twice the quantity necessary for all tests required to determine whether the active ingredient meets its established specifications, except for sterility and pyrogen testing. The retention time is as follows:

1. For an active ingredient in a drug product other than those described in paragraphs (a) (2) and (3) of this section, the reserve sample shall be retained for 1 year after the expiration date of the last lot of the drug product containing the active ingredient.

2. For an active ingredient in a radioactive drug product, except for non-radioactive reagent kits, the reserve sample shall be retained for
   i. Three months after the expiration date of the last lot of the drug product containing the active ingredient if the expiration dating period of the drug product is 30 days or less; or
   ii. Six months after the expiration date of the last lot of the drug product containing the active ingredient if the expiration dating period of the drug product is more than 30 days.

3. For an active ingredient in an OTC drug product that is exempt from bearing an expiration date under 211.137, the reserve sample shall be retained for 3 years after distribution of the last lot of the drug product containing the active ingredient.

b. An appropriately identified reserve sample that is representative of each lot or batch of drug product shall be retained and stored under conditions consistent with product labelling. The reserve sample shall be stored in the same immediate container-closure system in which the drug product is marketed or in one that has essentially the same characteristics. The reserve sample consists of at least twice the quantity necessary to perform all the required tests, except those for sterility and pyrogens. Except for those for drug products described in paragraph (b)(2) of this section, reserve samples from representative sample lots or batches selected by acceptable statistical procedures shall be examined visually at least once a year for evidence of deterioration unless visual examination would affect the integrity of the reserve sample. Any evidence of reserve sample deterioration shall be investigated in accordance with 211.192. The results of the examination shall be recorded and maintained with other stability data on the drug product. Reserve samples of compressed medical gases need not be retained. The retention time is as follows:

1. For a drug product other than those described in paragraphs (b) (2) and (3) of this section, the reserve sample shall be retained for 1 year after the expiration date of the drug product.
2. For a radioactive drug product, except for nonradioactive reagent kits, the reserve sample shall be retained for
    i. Three months after the expiration date of the drug product if the expiration dating period of the drug product is 30 days or less; or
    ii. Six months after the expiration date of the drug product if the expiration-dating period of the drug product is more than 30 days.
3. For an OTC drug product that is exempt for bearing an expiration date under 211.137, the reserve sample must be retained for 3 years after the lot or batch of drug product is distributed.

[48 FR 13025, Mar. 29, 1983, as amended at 60 FR 4091, Jan. 20, 1995]

Sec. 211.173. Laboratory animals

Animals used in testing components, in-process materials or drug products for compliance with established specifications shall be maintained and controlled in a manner that assures their suitability for their intended use. They shall be identified and adequate records shall be maintained showing the history of their use.

Sec. 211.176. Penicillin contamination

If a reasonable possibility exists that a non-penicillin drug product has been exposed to cross-contamination with penicillin, the non-penicillin drug product shall be tested for the presence of penicillin. Such drug product shall not be marketed if detectable levels are found when tested according to procedures specified in Procedures for Detecting and Measuring Penicillin Contamination in Drugs, which is incorporated by reference. Copies are available from the Division of Research and Testing (HFD-470), Center for Drug Evaluation and Research, Food and Drug Administration, 5100 Paint Branch Pkwy College Park, MD 20740, or available for inspection at the National Archives and Records Administration (NARA).

QCT-12.2

 Health Santé
Canada Canada

Canadä

S.4. CONTROL OF THE DRUG SUBSTANCE

S.4.1. SPECIFICATION

(Information in this section is not required for Phase I Clinical Trial Applications)

A summary of the specification for the drug substance should be provided. The specification is a list of tests, references to analytical procedures and acceptance criteria, which are numerical limits, ranges or other criteria for the tests described. This includes tests for description, identification, purity and potency as well as other tests specific to the drug substance.

The specification can be summarized according to the table in the Quality Overall Summary template including the tests, method types (including source) and acceptance criteria. The acceptance criteria should also be provided in the summary of the specification. The method type should indicate the kind of analytical procedure used (e.g., visual, IR, UV, HPLC, laser diffraction, etc.); and source refers to the origin of the analytical procedure (e.g., USP, Ph.Eur., BP, House, etc.).

Phase II Clinical Trial Applications

Specifications are considered interim as they are based on a limited number of development batches. A higher degree of flexibility will be allowed in specifications with sufficient scientific justification (refer to Section S.4.5—*Justification of Specification*).

Phase III Clinical Trial Applications

Specifications are expected to be reassessed prior to the Phase III application and reflect those intended for the marketing application, based on additional manufacturing experience and stability information.

S.4.2. ANALYTICAL PROCEDURES

(Information in this section is not required for Phase I Clinical Trial Applications)

Phase II and III Clinical Trial Applications

A brief description of the analytical methods used for the drug substance should be provided for all tests included in the drug substance specifications (e.g., method type, column size, etc.). Detailed descriptions of the step-by-step analytical procedures should not be submitted for clinical trial applications, but should be available upon request.

Unless modified, it is not necessary to provide descriptions of Schedule B compendial analytical procedures.

S.4.3. Validation of Analytical Procedures

(Information in this section not required for Phase I Clinical Trial Applications)

Phase II and III Clinical Trial Applications

The suitability of the analytical methods and a tabulated summary of the validation carried out should be provided (e.g., results or values for specificity, linearity, range, accuracy, precision, intermediate precision, limit of detection and limit of quantitation, where applicable). Complete validation reports should not be provided for clinical trial applications.

For substances that comply with a Schedule B monograph, reference to the monograph will be considered sufficient.

S.4.4. Batch Analyses

Description of batches and results of batch analyses should be provided.

The discussion of results should focus on observations noted for the various tests, rather than reporting comments such as "All tests meet specifications." This could include ranges of analytical results and any trends that were observed. For quantitative tests (e.g., as in individual and total impurity tests and potency tests), it should be ensured that *actual numerical results* are provided rather than vague statements such as "within limits" or "conforms." When reporting the analytical results it is important that the method used for each test be identified (including the type and the source).

Batch analysis results for the drug substance may be provided in either the Quality Overall Summary or by providing a copy of the Certificate of Analysis. The batch number, batch sizes and dates and sites of production should be stated for all batches.

Phase I Clinical Trial Applications

Analytical results from the batch(es) to be used in the proposed clinical trial should be provided.

Phase II Clinical Trial Applications

Analytical results from the batch(es) to be used in the proposed clinical trial should be provided. If batch analysis from the actual batches to be used in the proposed study are not available at the time of filing, results from representative batch(es) of drug substance may be provided as supporting data, with a commitment that the batch analysis for the specific lot to be used in that protocol will be submitted prior to dosing.

Phase III Clinical Trial Applications

Analytical results from the batch(es) to be used in the proposed clinical trial, or batches representative thereof, should be provided.

Note: For the purpose of this guidance document, a "representative batch" is defined as a batch of drug substance or drug product that is manufactured using the same formulation (for the drug product), method of manufacture and equipment, specifications and the same container closure system as the proposed clinical batch, with a similar batch size. All subsequent references in this guidance document to "representative batch" should be interpreted as per this definition.

S.4.5. JUSTIFICATION OF SPECIFICATION

(Information in this section is not required for Phase I Clinical Trial Applications)

The sponsor should ensure the specification includes all the tests and acceptance criteria appropriate for the drug substance, and that reasonable limits for impurities and residual solvents have been established. Acceptance criteria should be based on manufacturing experience, stability data and safety considerations.

S.6. CONTAINER CLOSURE SYSTEM

A description of the container closure system(s) should be provided, including the identity of materials of construction of each primary packaging component.

For non-functional secondary packaging components (e.g., those that do not provide additional protection), only a brief description should be provided. For functional secondary packaging components, additional information should be provided.

S.7. STABILITY

S.7.1. STABILITY SUMMARY AND CONCLUSIONS

The types of studies conducted, protocols used and the results of the studies should be summarized.

The tables in the Quality Overall Summary template can be used to summarize the information on the batches used in the stability studies. Full long-term stability data are not required at the time of filing, provided some preliminary stability data are available on the representative batches together with a commitment that the stability of the clinical trial samples or representative batches will be monitored according to the stability protocol until the retest period has been established.

The discussion of results should focus on observations noted for the various tests, rather than reporting comments such as "All tests meet specifications." This could include ranges of analytical results and any trends that were observed. For quantitative tests (e.g., as in individual and total degradation product tests and potency tests), it should be ensured that *actual numerical results* are provided rather than vague statements such as "within limits" or "conforms."

Available long-term and accelerated stability data for the drug substance should be provided at each stage of development to support its storage (conditions and retest period) and use in the manufacture of the drug product.

The proposed storage conditions and retest period (or shelf life, as appropriate) for the drug substance should be reported.

Stress Testing

Stress testing of the drug substance can help identify the likely degradation products, which can in turn help establish the degradation pathways, the intrinsic stability of the molecule and validate the stability indicating power of the analytical procedures used. The nature of the stress testing will depend on the individual drug substance and the type of drug product being developed.

S.7.2. STABILITY PROTOCOL AND STABILITY COMMITMENT

If full long-term stability data supporting the retest period are not available at the time of filing, provide a commitment that the stability of the clinical trial samples, or batches considered representative thereof, will be monitored according to the stability protocol. A summary of the stability protocol (in tabular format, summarizing frequency of testing, tests to be conducted, etc.) should be provided.

S.7.3. STABILITY DATA

Results of the stability studies (e.g., long-term studies, accelerated studies, stress conditions, etc.) should be presented in an appropriate format.

The actual stability results (i.e., raw data) used to support the clinical trial should be provided as a separate attachment. For quantitative tests (e.g., as in individual and total degradation product tests and potency tests), it should be ensured that the *actual numerical results* are provided rather than vague statements such as "within limits" or "conforms."

Phase II and III Clinical Trial Applications

In cases where analytical procedures are only used in stability studies (i.e., stability-indicating assay method) and were not summarized in 2.3.S.4, a brief description of the analytical procedure as well as a tabulated summary of validation information should be provided per the instructions in Sections S.4.2 and S.4.3.

P. DRUG PRODUCT

P.1. Description and Composition of the Drug Product

A description of the drug product and its composition should be provided. The information provided should include

(a) *Description of the dosage form*

The description of the dosage form should include the physical description, available strengths, release mechanism, as well as any other distinguishable characteristics (e.g., "The proposed drug product is available as oval, round, immediate-release, aqueous film-coated tablet in three strengths (5 mg, 10 mg, and 20 mg)").

(b) *Composition, that is, list of all components of the dosage form, their amount on a per unit basis (including overages, if any) and a reference to their quality standards (e.g., compendial monographs or manufacturer's specifications)*

The composition should express the quantity of each component on a per unit basis (e.g., mg per tablet, mg per mL, mg per vial, etc.) and percentage basis including a statement of the total weight or measure of the dosage unit. This should include all components used in the manufacturing process, regardless if they appear in the final drug product. If the drug product is formulated using an active moiety, then the composition for the active ingredient should be clearly indicated (e.g., "1 mg of active ingredient base = 1.075 mg active ingredient hydrochloride"). All overages should be clearly indicated (e.g., "contains 2% overage of the active pharmaceutical ingredient to compensate for manufacturing losses").

The components should be declared by their proper or common names, quality standards (e.g., USP, Ph.Eur., House, etc.) and, if applicable, their grades (e.g., "Microcrystalline Cellulose NF (PH 102)"). The function of each component (e.g., diluent/filler, binder, disintegrant, lubricant, glidant, granulating solvent, coating agent, anti-microbial preservative, etc.) should also be stated.

The qualitative composition should be provided for all proprietary components or blends (e.g., capsule shells, colouring blends, imprinting inks, etc.).

(c) *Description of reconstitution diluent(s), if applicable*

List all reconstitution solvents/diluents to be used in the proposed clinical study.

If the reconstitution solvents/diluents are manufactured in-house, a separate drug product section (e.g., Sections P.1 through P.8) should be completed for the chemistry and manufacturing information for the reconstitution solvents/diluents.

(d) Type of container closure system used for accompanying reconstitution diluents, if applicable

A brief description of the container closure system(s) used for the accompanying reconstitution diluent should be provided, if applicable (for commercially purchased diluents, provide information only if the primary packaging has been changed);

(e) Qualitative list of the components of the placebo samples used in the clinical trials, if different from the components listed in P.1(b)

P.4. CONTROL OF EXCIPIENTS

P.4.1. SPECIFICATIONS

This includes the specifications for all excipients, including those that do not appear in the final drug product (e.g., solvents). If the standard claimed for an excipient is a Schedule B compendial monograph, it is sufficient to state that the excipient is tested according to the requirements of that standard, rather than reproducing the specifications found in the compendial monograph.

If the standard claimed for an excipient is a non-Schedule B compendial monograph (e.g., House standard) or includes tests that are supplementary to those appearing in the Schedule B compendial monograph, a copy of the specifications for the excipient should be provided.

Confirmation should be provided that none of the excipients which appear in the drug product are prohibited for use in drugs by the Canadian *Food and Drug Regulations.*

For excipients which are filed with Health Canada as a Drug Master Files (DMF), a Letter of Access should be provided as an attachment. For more information, please refer to Health Canada's current guidance document on filing and referencing of DMF.

P.4.5. EXCIPIENTS OF HUMAN OR ANIMAL ORIGIN

For excipients of human or animal origin, information should be provided regarding adventitious agents (e.g., sources, specifications; description of the testing performed; viral safety data).

This information should include biological source, country of origin, manufacturer and a brief description of the suitability of use based on the proposed controls.

For gelatin for use in pharmaceuticals, supporting data should be provided which confirms that the gelatin is free of bovine spongiform encephalopathy (BSE)/transmissible spongiform encephalopathy (TSE). If the supplier of the gelatin has a DMF registered with Health Canada, a Letter of Access should be provided.

Supporting information for excipients of human or animal origin should be provided as a separate attachment.

P.4.6. NOVEL EXCIPIENTS

For excipient(s) used for the first time in a drug product or by a new route of administration, full details of manufacture, characterization and controls should be provided, with cross references to supporting safety data (non-clinical and/or clinical) using the relevant sections of the Quality Overall Summary according to the drug substance and/or drug product format.

P.5. CONTROL OF DRUG PRODUCT

P.5.1. SPECIFICATION(S)

(Information in this section is not required for Phase I Clinical Trial Applications)

A summary of the specification(s) for the drug product should be provided. The specification is a list of tests, references to analytical procedures and acceptance criteria, which are numerical limits, ranges or other criteria for the tests described. This includes tests for description, identification, purity and potency as well as other tests specific to the dosage form.

The specification(s) can be summarized according to Health Canada's Quality Overall Summary template including the tests, method types, sources, and acceptance criteria. The method type should indicate the kind of analytical procedure used (e.g., visual, IR, UV, HPLC, etc.); and the source refers to the origin of the analytical procedure (e.g., USP, BP, House, etc.).

Phase II Clinical Trial Applications

Specifications are considered interim as they are based on a limited number of development batches. A higher degree of flexibility will be allowed in specifications with sufficient scientific justification (Refer to Section P.5.6—*Justification of Specification*).

Phase III Clinical Trial Applications

Specifications are expected to be reassessed prior to the Phase III submission and reflect those intended for the marketing application, based on additional manufacturing experience and stability information.

P.5.2. ANALYTICAL PROCEDURES

(Information in this section is not required for Phase I Clinical Trial Applications)

Phase II and III Clinical Trial Applications

A brief description of the analytical methods used for the drug product should be provided for all tests included in the drug product specifications (e.g., reverse-phase HPLC, GC, etc.). Detailed descriptions of the step-by-step analytical procedures should not be submitted for Clinical Trial Applications, although this information should be available upon request.

Unless modified, it is not necessary to provide a copy of Schedule B compendial procedures.

P.5.3. VALIDATION OF ANALYTICAL PROCEDURES

(Information in this section is not required for Phase I Clinical Trial Applications)

Phase II and III Clinical Trial Applications

Suitability of the analytical methods and a tabulated summary of the validation information should be provided (i.e., results or values for specificity, linearity, range, accuracy, precision, robustness, limit of detection and limit of quantitation where applicable). Complete validation reports should not be submitted for Clinical Trial Applications, although this information should be available upon request.

For substances that comply with a Schedule B monograph, reference to the monograph will be considered sufficient for all Clinical Trial Applications.

P.5.4. BATCH ANALYSES

A description of batches and results of batch analyses should be provided.

The discussion of results should focus on observations noted for the various tests, rather than reporting comments such as "all tests meet specifications." This could include ranges of analytical results and any trends that were observed. For quantitative tests (e.g., as in individual and total degradation product tests and potency tests), it should be ensured that the *actual numerical* results are provided rather than vague statements such as "within limits" or "conforms." When reporting the analytical results it is important that the method used be identified (including the type and the source).

Batch analysis results for the drug product may be provided in either the Quality Overall Summary or by providing a copy of the Certificate of Analysis. In all cases, the batch numbers, batch sizes, dates and sites of production, and input drug substance batches should be provided.

Phase I Clinical Trial Applications

Analytical results from the batch(es) to be used in the proposed clinical trial should be provided.

Phase II Clinical Trial Applications

Analytical results from the batch(es) to be used in the proposed clinical trial should be provided. If batch analysis from the actual batches to be used in the proposed study are not available at the time of filing, results from representative batches of drug product may be provided as supporting data with a commitment that the batch analysis for the specific lot(s) to be used in that protocol will be submitted prior to dosing.

Phase III Clinical Trial Applications

Analytical results from the batch(es) to be used in the proposed clinical trial, or batch(es) considered representative thereof, should be provided.

P.5.5. CHARACTERIZATION OF IMPURITIES

Information on the characterization of impurities should be provided, if not previously summarized in Section S.3.2—Impurities.

This information includes degradation products (e.g., from the interaction of the drug substance with excipients or the container closure system), solvents in the manufacturing process for the drug product, and so on. The tables in the Quality Overall Summary template in Section S.3.2 can be used to summarize this information.

This section may also be used to report any new impurities found in the drug product during stress testing (e.g., photostability testing).

P.5.6. JUSTIFICATION OF SPECIFICATION(S)

(Information in this section is not required for Phase I Clinical Trial Applications)

The sponsor should ensure that the specification(s) includes all the tests and acceptance criteria appropriate for the drug product, and that reasonable limits for degradation products have been established. Acceptance criteria should be based on manufacturing experience, stability data and safety considerations. For impurities/degradation products which are unique to the drug product, acceptance criteria should be supported by appropriate toxicology and safety studies.

P.7. CONTAINER CLOSURE SYSTEM

A description of the container closure system(s) to be used in the clinical trial should be provided, including the materials of construction for each packaging component. This includes packaging components that

1. Are product contact surfaces
2. Are used as a protective barrier to help ensure stability or sterility
3. Are used for drug delivery
4. Are necessary to ensure drug product quality during transportation

For sterile products, details of washing, sterilization and depyrogenation should be submitted in this section.

For dosage forms that have a higher potential for interaction between filling and container closure system (e.g., parenteral, ophthalmic products, oral solutions), additional detail may be required.

P.8. STABILITY

P.8.1. STABILITY SUMMARY AND CONCLUSIONS

The types of studies conducted, protocols used and the results of the studies should be summarized.

The tables in the Quality Overall Summary template can be used to summarize the information on the batches used in the stability studies. Full long-term stability data are not required at the time of filing, provided some preliminary stability data are available on representative batches together with a commitment that the stability of the clinical trial samples or (representative batches) will be monitored according to the stability protocol until the shelf life of the drug product has been established with confidence.

The discussion of results should focus on observations noted for the various tests, rather than reporting comments such as "All tests meet specifications." This could include ranges of analytical results and any trends that were observed. For quantitative tests (e.g., as in individual and total degradation product tests and potency tests), it should be ensured that *actual numerical results* are provided rather than vague statements such as "within limits" or "conforms."

For sterile products, sterility should be reported at the beginning and end of shelf life. During development it is expected that sterility will be monitored on a routine basis (e.g., annual basis) until the shelf life has been determined with confidence. For parenteral products, sub-visible particulate matter should be reported at every test interval until a shelf life has been established. Bacterial endotoxins need only be reported at the initial test interval.

For drug products which are reconstituted or diluted prior to administration, stability and compatibility studies covering the entire in-use period should be provided. Furthermore, for products, which are diluted or reconstituted into a secondary container closure system (i.e., infusion kit), compatibility data should be submitted to support in-use conditions in that specific container closure.

Available long-term and accelerated stability data should be provided for the drug product at each stage of development to support its storage conditions and shelf-life.

Stress Testing

For certain drug products, stress testing of dosage forms may be appropriate to assess the potential for changes in physical and/or chemical properties of the drug product. The nature of the stress testing will depend on the type of drug product being developed.

Proposed Storage Conditions and Shelf Life

The proposed storage conditions with suitable tolerances (e.g., a temperature range with upper and lower criteria) and shelf life for the drug product should be provided. Alternative storage conditions may be acceptable with supporting scientific data.

Based on the results of the stability evaluation, other storage precautions may be warranted (e.g., "Do not refrigerate," "Protect from light," "Protect from moisture").

P.8.2. STABILITY PROTOCOL AND STABILITY COMMITMENT

If full long-term stability data supporting the proposed shelf life are not available at the time of filing, provide a commitment that the stability of the clinical trial samples, or samples considered representative of the clinical batches, will be monitored throughout the duration of the clinical trial. A summary of the stability protocol (e.g., tabular format, summarizing frequency of testing, tests to be conducted, etc.) should be provided.

P.8.3. STABILITY DATA

Results of the stability studies (e.g., long-term and accelerated studies) should be presented in an appropriate format.

The actual stability results (i.e., raw data) used to support the clinical trial should be provided as an attachment. For quantitative tests (e.g., as in individual and total degradation product tests and potency tests), it should be ensured that the *actual numerical results* are provided rather than vague statements such as "within limits" or "conforms."

Phase II and III Clinical Trial Applications

In cases where analytical procedures are only used in stability studies (i.e., stability indicating assay method) and were not previously summarized, details of the analytical procedure as well as a tabulated summary of validation information should be provided per the instructions in Sections P.5.2 and P.5.3.

CLV-12.3

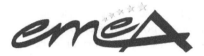

EUROPEAN MEDICINES AGENCY

Directive 2004/9/EC of the European Parliament and of the Council of 11 February 2004 on the inspection and verification of good laboratory practice (GLP)
(Codified version)
(Text with EEA relevance)

THE EUROPEAN PARLIAMENT AND THE COUNCIL OF THE EUROPEAN UNION

Having regard to the Treaty establishing the European Community, and in particular Article 95 thereof,

Having regard to the proposal from the Commission,

Having regard to the opinion of the European Economic and Social Committee (1),

Acting in accordance with the procedure laid down in Article 251 of the Treaty (2),

whereas:

1. Council Directive 88/320/EEC of 7 June 1988 on the inspection and verification of Good Laboratory Practice (GLP) (3) has been significantly amended several times. In the interests of clarity and rationality the said Directive should be codified.

2. The application of standardized organizational processes and conditions under which laboratory studies are planned, performed, recorded and reported for the non-clinical testing of chemicals for the protection of man, animals and the environment, hereinafter referred to as "good laboratory practice" (GLP), contributes to the reassurance of Member States as to the quality of the test data generated.

3. In Annex 2 to its Decision of 12 May 1981 on the mutual acceptance of data in the assessment of chemicals, the Council of the Organisation for

Economic Cooperation and Development (OECD) adopted principles of good laboratory practice which are accepted within the Community and are specified in the European Parliament and Council Directive 2004/10/EC of 11 February 2004 on the harmonization of laws, regulations and administrative provisions relating to the application of the principles of good laboratory practice and the verification of their applications for tests on chemical substances.

4. In the conduct of tests on chemicals, it is desirable that specialist manpower and testing laboratory resources should not be wasted owing to the need to duplicate tests because of differences in laboratory practices from one Member State to another. This applies especially for animal protection which requires that the number of experiments on animals be restricted in accordance with Council Directive 86/609/EEC of 24 November 1986 on the approximation of laws, regulations and administrative provisions of the Member States regarding the protection of animals used for experimental and other scientific purposes (5). Mutual recognition of the results of tests obtained using standard and recognized methods is an essential condition for reducing the number of experiments in this area.

5. However, in order to ensure that test data generated by laboratories in one Member State are also recognized by other Member States, it is necessary to provide for a harmonized system for study audit and inspection of laboratories to ensure that they are working under GLP conditions.

6. Member States should designate the authorities responsible for carrying out monitoring on compliance with GLP.

7. A committee, the members of which will be appointed by the Member States, would be of assistance to the Commission in the technical application of this Directive and would cooperate in its efforts to encourage the free movement of goods through the mutual recognition by Member States of procedures for monitoring compliance with GLP. The Committee set up by Council Directive 67/548/EEC of 27 June 1967 on the approximation of laws, regulations and administrative provisions relating to the classification, packaging and labelling of dangerous substances (6) should be used for this purpose.

8. That Committee may assist the Commission not only in the application of this Directive but also in contributing to the exchange of information and experience in this field.

9. The measures necessary for the implementation of this Directive should be adopted in accordance with Council Decision 1999/468/EC of 28 June 1999 laying down the procedures for the exercise of implementing powers conferred on the Commission (7).

10. This Directive should be without prejudice to the obligations of the Member States concerning the time-limits for transposition of the Directives set out in:

ANNEX II, PART B

HAVE ADOPTED THIS DIRECTIVE

Article 1

1. This Directive shall apply to the inspection and verification of the organizational processes and the conditions under which laboratory studies are planned, performed, recorded and reported for the non-clinical testing, carried out in accordance with the rules and regulations, of all chemicals (e.g., cosmetics, industrial chemicals, medicinal products, food additives, animal feed additives, pesticides) in order to assess the effect of such products on man, animals and the environment.
2. For the purposes of this Directive, "good laboratory practice" (GLP), shall mean laboratory practice conducted in accordance with the principles set out in Directive 2004/10/EC.
3. This Directive does not concern the interpretation and evaluation of test results.

Article 2

1. Using the procedure laid down in Article 3, Member States shall verify the compliance with GLP of any testing laboratory within their territory claiming to use GLP in the conduct of tests on chemicals.
2. Where the provisions of paragraph 1 have been complied with, and the results of the inspection and verification are satisfactory, the Member State in question may provide endorsement of a claim by a laboratory that it and the tests that it carries out comply with GLP, using the formula "Assessment of conformity with GLP according to Directive 2004/9/EC on ... (date)."

Article 3

1. Member States shall designate the authorities responsible for the inspection of laboratories within their territories and for the audit of studies carried out by laboratories to assess compliance with GLP.
2. The authorities referred to in paragraph 1 shall inspect the laboratory and audit the studies in accordance with the provisions laid down in Annex I.

Article 4

1. Each year, Member States shall draw up a report relating to the implementation of GLP within their territory. This report shall contain a list of laboratories inspected, the date on which such inspection was carried out and a brief summary of the conclusions of the inspections.
2. The reports shall be forwarded to the Commission each year, not later than 31 March. The Commission shall communicate them to the Committee referred to in Article 7(1). The Committee may request information in addition to those elements mentioned in paragraph 1 of this Article.

3. Member States shall ensure that commercially sensitive and other confidential information to which they gain access as a result of GLP compliance monitoring activities is made available only to the Commission, to national regulatory and designated authorities and to a laboratory or study sponsor directly concerned with a particular inspection or study audit.
4. The names of laboratories subject to inspection by a designated authority, their GLP compliance status and the dates upon which laboratory inspections or study audits have been conducted shall not be considered to be confidential.

Article 5

1. Without prejudice to Article 6, the results of laboratory inspections and study audits on GLP compliance carried out by a Member State shall be binding on the other Member States.
2. Where a Member State considers that a laboratory within its territory claiming GLP compliance does not in fact comply with GLP to the extent that the integrity or authenticity of the studies it performs might be compromised, it shall forthwith inform the Commission. The Commission shall inform the other Member States.

Article 6

1. Where a Member State has sufficient reason to believe that a laboratory in another Member State claiming GLP compliance has not carried out a test in accordance with GLP, it may request further information from that Member State and in particular may request a study audit, possibly in conjunction with a new inspection. Should it not be possible for the Member States concerned to reach agreement, the Member States in question shall immediately inform the other Member States and the Commission, giving reasons for their decision.
2. The Commission shall examine as soon as possible the reasons put forward by the Member States within the Committee referred to in Article 7(1); it shall then take the appropriate measures in accordance with procedure referred to in Article 7(2). It may in this connection ask for expert opinions from the designated authorities in the Member States.
3. If the Commission considers that amendments to this Directive are necessary in order to resolve the matters referred to in paragraph 1, it shall initiate the procedure referred to in Article 7(2) with a view to adopting those amendments.

Article 7

1. The Commission shall be assisted by the Committee set up in Article 29 of Directive 67/548/EEC, hereinafter "the Committee."
2. Where reference is made to this paragraph, Articles 5 and 7 of Decision 1999/468/EC shall apply, having regard to the provisions of Article 8 thereof.

3. The period laid down in Article 5(6) of Decision 1999/468/EC shall be set at three months.

4. The Committee shall adopt its Rules of Procedure.

Article 8

1. The Committee may examine any question which is referred to it by its chairman either on his own initiative or at the request of a representative of a Member State, concerning the implementation of this Directive and in particular regarding:

   - Cooperation between the authorities designated by the Member States in technical and administrative matters arising from the implementation of GLP, and
   - The exchange of information on the training of inspectors.
   - The amendments necessary for the adaptation of the formula referred to in Article 2(2) and of Annex I to take account of technical progress shall be adopted in accordance with the procedure referred to in Article 7(2).

Article 9

Directive 88/320/EEC is hereby repealed, without prejudice to the obligations of the Member States concerning the time limits for transposition of the said Directives as set out in Annex II, Part B.

References made to the repealed Directive shall be construed as being made to this Directive and shall be read in accordance with the correlation table in Annex III.

Article 10

This Directive shall enter into force on the 20th day following that of its publication in the *Official Journal* of the European Union.

Article 11

This Directive is addressed to the Member States.

Done at Strasbourg, 11 February 2004.
For the European Parliament
The President
P. Cox
For the Council
The President
M. McDowell

1. OJ C 85, 8.4.2003, p. 137.
2. Opinion of the European Parliament of 1 July 2003 (not yet published in the *Official Journal*) and Decision of the Council of 20 January 2004.

3. OJ L 145, 11.6.1988, p. 35. Directive as last amended by Regulation (EC) No 1882/2003 of the European Parliament and of the Council (OJ L 284, 31.10.2003, p. 1).

4. See page 44 of this *Official Journal*.

5. OJ L 358, 18.12.1986, p. 1.

6. OJ 196, 16.8.1967, p. 1. Directive as last amended by Council Regulation (EC) No 807/2003 (OJ L 122, 16.5.2003, p. 36).

7. OJ L 184, 17.7.1999, p. 23.

ANNEX I

The provisions for the inspection and verification of GLP which are contained in Parts A and B are those contained in Annexes I (Guides for compliance monitoring procedures for good laboratory practice) and II (Guidance for the conduct of test facility inspections and study audits), respectively of the OECD Council Decision-Recommendation on compliance with principles of good laboratory practice (C(89)87(Final)) of 2 October 1989 as revised by the OECD Council Decision amending the Annexes to the Council Decision-Recommendation on compliance with principles of good laboratory practice of 9 March 1995 (C(95)8(Final)).

PART A REVISED GUIDES FOR COMPLIANCE MONITORING PROCEDURES FOR GLP

To facilitate the mutual acceptance of test data generated for submission to Regulatory Authorities of the OECD member countries, harmonization of the procedures adopted to monitor GLP compliance, as well as comparability of their quality and rigour, are essential. The aim of this part of this Annex is to provide detailed practical guidance to the Member States on the structure, mechanisms and procedures they should adopt when establishing national GLP compliance monitoring programmes so that these programmes may be internationally acceptable.

It is recognized that Member States will adopt GLP principles and establish compliance monitoring procedures according to national legal and administrative practices, and according to priorities they give to, for example the scope of initial and subsequent coverage concerning categories of chemicals and types of testing. Since Member States may establish more than one GLP Monitoring Authority due to their legal framework for chemicals control, more than one GLP compliance programme may be established. The guidance set forth in the following paragraphs concerns each of these Authorities and compliance programmes, as appropriate.

Definitions of Terms

The definitions of terms in the OECD principles of good laboratory practice adopted in Article 1 of Directive 2004/10/EC of the European Parliament and of the Council are applicable to this part of this Annex. In addition, the following definitions apply:

- GLP principles: principles of good laboratory practice that are consistent with the OECD principles of good laboratory practice as adopted in Article 1 of Directive 2004/10/EC.
- GLP compliance monitoring: the periodic inspection of test facilities and/or auditing of studies for the purpose of verifying adherence to GLP principles.
- (national) GLP compliance programme: the particular scheme established by a Member State to monitor GLP compliance by test facilities within its territories, by means of inspections and study audits.
- (national) GLP Monitoring Authority: a body established within a Member State with responsibility for monitoring the GLP compliance of test facilities within its territories and for discharging other such functions related to GLP as may be nationally determined. It is understood that more than one such body may be established in a Member State.
- Test facility inspection: an on-site examination of the test facility's procedures and practices to assess the degree of compliance with GLP principles. During inspections, the management structures and operational procedures of the test facility are examined, key technical personnel are interviewed, and the quality and integrity of data generated by the facility are assessed and reported.
- Study audit: a comparison of raw data and associated records with the interim or final report in order to determine whether the raw data have been accurately reported, to determine whether testing was carried out in accordance with the study plan and standard operating procedures (SOPs), to obtain additional information not provided in the report, and to establish whether practices were employed in the development of data that would impair their validity.
- Inspector: a person who performs the test facility inspections and study audits on behalf of the (national) GLP Monitoring Authority.
- GLP compliance status: the level of adherence of a test facility to the GLP principles as assessed by the (national) GLP Monitoring Authority.
- Regulatory Authority: a national body with legal responsibility for aspects of the control of chemicals.

Components of good laboratory practice compliance monitoring procedures:

Administration

A (national) GLP compliance programme should be the responsibility of a properly constituted, legally identifiable body adequately staffed and working within a defined administrative framework.

Member States should:

- Ensure that the (national) GLP Monitoring Authority is directly responsible for an adequate "team" of inspectors having the necessary technical/scientific expertise or is ultimately responsible for such a team.
- Publish documents relating to the adoption of GLP principles within their territories.
- Publish documents providing details of the (national) GLP compliance programme, including information on the legal or administrative framework within which the programme operates and references to published acts, normative documents (e.g., regulations, codes of practice), inspection manuals, guidance notes, periodicity of inspections and/or criteria for inspection schedules, and so on.
- Maintain records of test facilities inspected (and their GLP compliance status) and of studies audited for both national and international purposes.

Confidentiality

(National) GLP Monitoring Authorities will have access to commercially valuable information and, on occasion, may even need to remove commercially sensitive documents from a test facility or refer to them in detail in their reports.
Member States should:

- Make provision for the maintenance of confidentiality, not only by Inspectors but also by any other persons who gain access to confidential information as a result of GLP compliance monitoring activities.
- Ensure that, unless all commercially sensitive and confidential information has been excised, reports of test facility inspections and study audits are made available only to Regulatory Authorities and, where appropriate, to the test facilities inspected or concerned with study audits and/or to study sponsors.

Personnel and Training

(National) GLP Monitoring Authorities should:

- Ensure that an adequate number of inspectors is available.

The number of inspectors required will depend on:

a. The number of test facilities involved in the (national) GLP compliance programme;
b. The frequency with which the GLP compliance status of the test facilities is to be assessed;
c. The number and complexity of the studies undertaken by those test facilities;

d. The number of special inspections or audits requested by Regulatory Authorities,
   - Ensure that inspectors are adequately qualified and trained.

Inspectors should have qualifications and practical experience in the range of scientific disciplines relevant to the testing of chemicals. (National) GLP Monitoring Authorities should:

a. Ensure that arrangements are made for the appropriate training of GLP inspectors, having regard to their individual qualifications and experience;
b. Encourage consultations, including joint training activities where necessary, with the staff of (national) GLP Monitoring Authorities in other OECD member countries in order to promote international harmonization in the interpretation and application of GLP principles, and in the monitoring of compliance with such principles,
   - Ensure that inspectorate personnel, including experts under contract, have no financial or other interests in the test facilities inspected, the studies audited or the firms sponsoring such studies,
   - Provide inspectors with a suitable means of identification (e.g., an identity card).

Inspectors may be:

- On the permanent staff of the (national) GLP Monitoring Authority,
- On the permanent staff of a body separate from the (national) GLP Monitoring Authority, or
- Employed on contract, or in another way, by the (national) GLP Monitoring Authority to perform test facility inspections or study audits.

In the latter two cases, the (national) GLP Monitoring Authority should have ultimate responsibility for determining the GLP compliance status of test facilities and the quality/acceptability of a study audit, and for taking any action based on the results of test facility inspections or study audits which may be necessary.

(National) GLP compliance programmes:

GLP compliance monitoring is intended to ascertain whether test facilities have implemented GLP principles for the conduct of studies and are capable of assuring that the resulting data are of adequate quality. As indicated above, Member States should publish the details of their (national) GLP compliance programmes. Such information should, *inter alia*:

- Define the scope and extent of the programme.

A (national) GLP compliance programme may cover only a limited range of chemicals, for example, industrial chemicals, pesticides, pharmaceuticals, and so on, or may include all chemicals. The scope of the monitoring for compliance should be defined, both with respect to the categories of chemicals and to the types of tests subject to it, for example, physical, chemical, toxicological and/or ecotoxicological,

- Provide an indication as to the mechanism whereby test facilities enter the programme.

The application of GLP principles to health and environmental safety data generated for regulatory purposes may be mandatory. A mechanism should be available whereby test facilities may have their compliance with GLP principles monitored by the appropriate (national) GLP Monitoring Authority,

- Provide information on categories of test facility inspections/study audits.

A (national) GLP compliance programme should include:

a. Provision for test facility inspections. These inspections include both a general test facility inspection and a study audit of one or more on-going or completed studies;
b. Provisions for special test facility inspections/study audits at the request of a Regulatory Authority, for example, prompted by a query arising from the submission of data to a Regulatory Authority,
  - Define the powers of inspectors for entry into test facilities and their access to data held by test facilities (including specimens, SOPs, other documentation, etc.).

While inspectors will not normally wish to enter test facilities against the will of the facility's management, circumstances may arise where test facility entry and access to data are essential to protect public health or the environment. The powers available to the (national) GLP Monitoring Authority in such cases should be defined,

- Describe the test facility inspection and study audit procedures for verification of GLP compliance.

The documentation should indicate the procedures which will be used to examine both the organizational processes and the conditions under which studies are planned, performed, monitored and recorded. Guidance for such procedures is available in part B of this Annex,

- Describe actions that may be taken as follow-up test facility inspections and study audits.

Follow-up to test facility inspections and study audits.

When a test facility inspection or study audit has been completed, the inspector should prepare a written report of the findings.

Member States should take action where deviations from GLP principles are found during or after a test facility inspection or study audit. The appropriate actions should be described in documents from the (national) GLP Monitoring Authority.

If a test facility inspection or study audit reveals only minor deviations from GLP principles, the facility should be required to correct such minor deviations. The inspector may need, at an appropriate time, to return to the facility to verify that corrections have been introduced.

Where no, or where only minor deviations have been found, the (national) GLP Monitoring Authority may:

- Issue a statement that the test facility has been inspected and found to be operating in compliance with GLP principles. The date of the inspections and, if appropriate, the categories of test inspected in the test facility at that time should be included. Such statements may be used to provide information to (national) GLP Monitoring Authorities in other OECD member countries, and/or
- Provide the Regulatory Authority which requested a study audit with a detailed report of the findings.

Where serious deviations are found, the action taken by (national) GLP Monitoring Authorities will depend on the particular circumstances of each case and the legal or administrative provisions under which GLP compliance monitoring has been established within their countries. Actions which may be taken include, but are not limited to, the following:

- Issuance of a statement, giving details of the inadequacies or faults found which might affect the validity of studies conducted in the test facility.
- Issuance of a recommendation to a Regulatory Authority that a study be rejected.
- Suspension of test facility inspections or study audits of a test facility and, for example and where administratively possible, removal of the test facility from the (national) GLP compliance programme or from any existing list or register of test facilities subject to GLP test facility inspections.
- Requiring that a statement detailing the deviations be attached to specific study reports.
- Action through the courts, where warranted by circumstances and where legal/administrative procedures so permit.

Appeals Procedures

Problems, or differences of opinion, between inspectors and test facility management will normally be resolved during the course of a test facility inspection or study audit. However, it may not always be possible for agreement to be reached. A procedure should exist whereby a test facility may make representations relating to the outcome of a test facility inspection or study audit for GLP compliance monitoring and/or relating to the action the GLP Monitoring Authority proposes to take thereon.

PART B REVISED GUIDANCE FOR THE CONDUCT OF TEST FACILITY INSPECTIONS AND STUDY AUDITS

Introduction

The purpose of this part of this Annex is to provide guidance for the conduct of test facility inspections and study audits which would be mutually acceptable to OECD member countries. It is principally concerned with test facility inspections, an activity which occupies much of the time of GLP inspectors. A test facility inspection will usually include a study audit or review as a part of the inspection, but study audits will also have to be conducted from time to time at the request, for example, of a Regulatory Authority. General guidance for the conduct of study audits will be found at the end of this Annex.

Test facility inspections are conducted to determine the degree of conformity of test facilities and studies with GLP principles and to determine the integrity of data to assure that resulting data are of adequate quality for assessment and decision-making by national Regulatory Authorities. They result in reports which describe the degree of adherence of a test facility to the GLP principles. Test facility inspections should be conducted on a regular, routine basis to establish and maintain records of the GLP compliance status of test facilities.

Further clarification of many of the points in this part of this Annex may be obtained by referring to the OECD consensus documents on GLP (on, e.g., the roles and responsibilities of the study director).

Definitions of Terms

The definitions of terms in the OECD principles of GLP adopted in Article 1 of Directive 2004/10/EC and in Part A of this Annex are applicable to this part of this Annex.

Test Facility Inspections

Inspections for compliance with GLP principles may take place in any test facility generating health or environmental safety data for regulatory purposes. Inspectors may be required to audit data relating to the physical, chemical, toxicological or ecotoxicological properties of a substance or preparation. In some cases, inspectors may need assistance from experts in particular disciplines.

The wide diversity of facilities (in terms both of physical layout and management structure), together with the variety of types of studies encountered by inspectors, means that the inspectors must use their own judgment to assess the degree and extent of compliance with GLP principles. Nevertheless, inspectors should strive for a consistent approach in evaluating whether, in the case of a particular test facility or study, an adequate level of compliance with each GLP principle has been achieved.

In the following sections, guidance is provided on the various aspects of the testing facility, including its personnel and procedures, which are likely to be examined by inspectors. In each section, there is a statement of purpose, as well as an illustrative list of specific items which could be considered during the course of a test facility inspection. These lists are not meant to be comprehensive and should not be taken as such.

Inspectors should not concern themselves with the scientific design of the study or the interpretation of the findings of studies with respect to risks for human health or the environment. These aspects are the responsibilities of those Regulatory Authorities to which the data are submitted for regulatory purposes.

Test facility inspections and study audits inevitably disturb the normal work in a facility. Inspectors should therefore carry out their work in a carefully planned way and, so far as practicable, respect the wishes of the management of the test facility as to the timing of visits to certain sections of the facility.

Inspectors will, while conducting test facility inspections and study audits, have access to confidential, commercially valuable information. It is essential that they ensure that such information is seen by authorized personnel only. Their responsibilities in this respect will have been established within their (national) GLP compliance monitoring programme.

Inspection Procedures

Pre-inspection

Purpose: to familiarize the inspector with the facility which is about to be inspected in respect of management structure, physical layout of buildings and range of studies.

Prior to conducting a test facility inspection or study audit, inspectors should familiarize themselves with the facility which is to be visited. Any existing information on the facility should be reviewed. This may include previous inspection reports, the layout of the facility, organization charts, study reports, protocols and curricula vitae (CVs) of personnel. Such documents would provide information on:

- The type, size and layout of the facility
- The range of studies likely to be encountered during the inspection
- The management structure of the facility

Inspectors should note, in particular, any deficiencies from previous test facility inspections. Where no previous test facility inspections have been conducted, a pre-inspection visit can be made to obtain relevant information.

Test facilities may be informed of the date and time of inspector's arrival, the objective of their visit and the length of time they expect to be on the premises. This could allow the test facility to ensure that the appropriate personnel and documentation are available. In cases where particular documents or records are to be examined, it may be useful to identify these to the test facility in advance of the visit so that they will be immediately available during the test facility inspection.

Starting Conference

Purpose: to inform the management and staff of the facility of the reason for the test facility inspection or study audit that is about to take place, and to identify the facility areas, study(ies) selected for audit, documents and personnel likely to be involved.

The administrative and practical details of a test facility inspection or study audit should be discussed with the management of the facility at the start of the visit. At the starting conference, inspectors should:

- Outline the purpose and scope of the visit
- Describe the documentation which will be required for the test facility inspection, such as lists of on-going and completed studies, study plans, standard operating procedures, study reports, and so on. Access to and, if necessary, arrangements for the copying of relevant documents should be agreed on at this time
- Clarify or request information as to the management structure (organization) and personnel of the facility
- Request information as to the conduct of studies not subject to GLP principles in the areas of the test facility where GLP studies are being conducted
- Make an initial determination as to the parts of the facility to be covered during the test facility inspection
- Describe the documents and specimens that will be needed for on-going or completed study(ies) selected for study audit
- Indicate that a closing conference will be held at the completion of the inspection

Before proceeding further with a test facility inspection, it is advisable for the inspector(s) to establish contact with the facility's quality assurance (QA) unit.

As a general rule, when inspecting a facility, inspectors will find it helpful to be accompanied by a member of the QA unit.

Inspectors may wish to request that a room be set aside for examination of documents and other activities.

Organization and Personnel

Purpose: to determine whether the test facility has sufficient qualified personnel, staff resources and support services for the variety and number of studies undertaken; the organizational structure is appropriate, and management has established a policy regarding training and staff health surveillance appropriate to the studies undertaken in the facility.

The management should be asked to produce certain documents, such as:

- Floor plans
- Facility management and scientific organization charts
- CVs of personnel involved in the type(s) of studies selected for the study audit
- List(s) of on-going and completed studies with information on the type of study, initiation/completion dates, test system, method of application of test substance and name of study director
- Staff health surveillance policies
- Staff job descriptions and staff training programmes and records
- An index to the facility's standard operating procedures (SOPs)
- Specific SOPs as related to the studies or procedures being inspected or audited
- List(s) of the study directors and sponsors associated with the study(ies) being audited

The inspector should check, in particular:

- Lists of on-going and completed studies to ascertain the level of work being undertaken by the test facility
- The identity and qualifications of the study director(s), the head of the quality assurance unit and other personnel
- Existence of SOPs for all relevant areas of testing

Quality Assurance Programme

Purpose: to determine whether the mechanisms used to assure management that studies are conducted in accordance with GLP principles are adequate.

The head of the QA unit should be asked to demonstrate the systems and methods for QA inspection and monitoring of studies, and the system for recording observations made during QA monitoring. Inspectors should check:

- The qualifications of the head of QA, and of all QA staff
- That the QA unit functions independently from the staff involved in the studies
- How the QA unit schedules and conducts inspections, how it monitors identified critical phases in a study, and what resources are available for QA inspections and monitoring activities
- That where studies are of such short duration that monitoring of each study is impracticable, arrangements exist for monitoring on a sample basis

- The extent and depth of QA monitoring during the practical phases of the study
- The extent and depth of QA monitoring of routine test facility operation
- The QA procedure for checking the final report to ensure its agreement with the raw data
- That management receives reports from QA concerning problems likely to affect the quality or integrity of a study
- The actions taken by QA when deviations are found
- The QA role, if any, if studies or parts of studies are done in contract laboratories
- The part played, if any, by QA in the review, revision and updating of SOPs

Facilities

Purpose: to determine if the test facility, whether indoor or outdoor, is of suitable size, design and location to meet the demands of the studies being undertaken.

The inspector should check that:

- The design enables an adequate degree of separation so that, for example, test substances, animals, diets, pathological specimens, and so on of one study cannot be confused with those of another
- Environmental control and monitoring procedures exist and function adequately in critical areas, for example, animal and other biological test systems rooms, test substance storage areas, laboratory areas
- The general housekeeping is adequate for the various facilities and that there are, if necessary, pest control procedures

Care, Housing and Containment of Biological Test Systems

Purpose: to determine whether the test facility, if engaged in studies using animals or other biological test systems, has support facilities and conditions for their care, housing and containment, adequate to prevent stress and other problems which could affect the test system and hence the quality of data.

A test facility may be carrying out studies which require a diversity of animal or plant species as well as microbial or other cellular or sub-cellular systems. The type of test systems being used will determine the aspects relating to care, housing or containment that the inspector will monitor. Using his judgment, the inspector will check, according to the test systems, that:

- There are facilities adequate for the test systems used and for testing needs
- There are arrangements to quarantine animals and plants being introduced into the facility and that these arrangements are working satisfactorily

- There are arrangements to isolate animals (or other elements of a test system, if necessary) known to be, or suspected of being, diseased or carriers of disease
- There is adequate monitoring and record-keeping of health, behaviour or other aspects, as appropriate to the test system
- The equipment for maintaining the environmental conditions required for each test system is adequate, well maintained, and effective
- Animal cages, racks, tanks and other containers, as well as accessory equipment, are kept sufficiently clean
- Analyses to check environmental conditions and support systems are carried out as required
- Facilities exist for removal and disposal of animal waste and refuse from the test systems and that these are operated so as to minimize vermin infestation, odours, disease hazards and environmental contamination
- Storage areas are provided for animal feed or equivalent materials for all test systems; that these areas are not used for the storage of other materials such as test substances, pest control chemicals or disinfectants, and that they are separate from areas in which animals are housed or other biological test systems are kept
- Stored feed and bedding are protected from deterioration by adverse environmental conditions, infestation or contamination

Apparatus, Materials, Reagents and Specimens

Purpose: to determine whether the test facility has suitably located, operational apparatus in sufficient quantity and of adequate capacity to meet the requirements of the tests being conducted in the facility and that the materials, reagents and specimens are properly labelled, used and stored.

The inspector should check that:

- Apparatus is clean and in good working order
- Records have been kept of operation, maintenance, verification, calibration and validation of measuring equipment and apparatus (including computerized systems)
- Materials and chemical reagents are properly labelled and stored at appropriate temperatures and that expiry dates are not being ignored. Labels for reagents should indicate their source, identity and concentration and/or other pertinent information
- Specimens are well identified by test system, study, nature and date of collection
- Apparatus and materials used do not alter to any appreciable extent the test systems

Test Systems

Purpose: to determine whether adequate procedures exist for the handling and control of the variety of test systems required by the studies undertaken in the facility, for example, chemical and physical systems, cellular and microbic systems, plants or animals.

Physical and Chemical Systems

The inspector should check that:

- Where required by study plans, the stability of test and reference substances was determined and that the reference substances specified in test plans were used
- In automated systems, data generated as graphs, recorder traces or computer print-outs are documented as raw data and archived

Biological Test Systems

Taking account of the relevant aspects referred to above relating to care, housing or containment of biological test systems, the inspector should check that:

- Test systems are as specified in study plans
- Test systems are adequately and, if necessary and appropriate, uniquely identified throughout the study, and that records exist regarding receipt of the test systems and document fully the number of test systems received, used, replaced or discarded
- Housing or containers of test systems are properly identified with all the necessary information
- There is an adequate separation of studies being conducted on the same animal species (or the same biological test systems) but with different substances
- There is an adequate separation of animal species (and other biological test systems) either in space or in time
- The biological test system environment is as specified in the study plan or in SOPs for aspects such as temperature, or light/dark cycles
- The recording of the receipt, handling, housing or containment, care and health evaluation is appropriate to the test systems
- Written records are kept of examination, quarantine, morbidity, mortality, behaviour, diagnosis and treatment of animal and plant test systems or other similar aspects as appropriate to each biological test system
- There are provisions for the appropriate disposal of test systems at the end of tests

Test and Reference Substances

Purpose: to determine whether the test facility has procedures designed (i) to ensure that the identity, potency, quantity and composition of test and reference substances are in accordance with their specifications, and (ii) to properly receive and store test and reference substances.

The inspector should check that:

- There are written records on the receipt (including identification of the person responsible), and for the handling, sampling, usage and storage of tests and reference substances
- Test and reference substances containers are properly labelled
- Storage conditions are appropriate to preserve the concentration, purity and stability of the test and reference substances
- There are written records on the determination of identity, purity, composition, stability, and for the prevention of contamination of test and reference substances, where applicable
- There are procedures for the determination of the homogeneity and stability of mixtures containing test and reference substances, where applicable
- Containers holding mixtures (or dilutions) of the test and reference substances are labelled and that records are kept of the homogeneity and stability of their contents, where applicable
- When the test is of longer than four weeks duration, samples from each batch of test and reference substances have been taken for analytical purposes and that they have been retained for an appropriate time
- Procedures for mixing substances are designed to prevent errors in identification or cross-contamination

Standard Operating Procedures

Purpose: to determine whether the test facility has written SOPs relating to all the important aspects of its operations, considering that one of the most important management techniques for controlling facility operations is the use of written SOPs. These relate directly to the routine elements of tests conducted by the test facility.

The inspector should check that:

- Each test facility area has immediately available relevant, authorized copies of SOPs
- Procedures exist for revision and updating of SOPs
- Any amendments or changes to SOPs have been authorized and dated
- Historical files of SOPs are maintained
- SOPs are available for, but not necessarily limited to, the following activities:
    i.   Receipt; determination of identity, purity, composition and stability; labelling; handling; sampling; usage; and storage of test and reference substances
    ii. Use, maintenance, cleaning, calibration and validation of measuring apparatus, computerized systems and environmental control equipment
    iii. Preparation of reagents and dosing formulations

    iv. Record-keeping, reporting, storage and retrieval of records and reports

    v. Preparation and environmental control of areas containing the test systems

    vi. Receipt, transfer, location, characterization, identification and care of test systems

    vii. Handling of the test systems before, during and at the termination of the study

    viii. Disposal of test systems

    ix. Use of pest control and cleaning agents

    x. Quality assurance programme operations

Performance of the Study

Purpose: to verify that written study plans exist and that the plans and the conduct of the study are in accordance with GLP principles.

The inspector should check that:

- The study plan was signed by the study director
- Any amendments to the study plan were signed and dated by the study director
- The date of the agreement to the study plan by the sponsor was recorded (where applicable)
- Measurements, observations and examinations were in accordance with the study plan and relevant SOPs
- The results of these measurements, observations and examinations were recorded directly, promptly, accurately and legibly and were signed (or initialled) and dated
- Any changes in the raw data, including data stored in computers, did not obscure previous entries, included the reason for the change and identified the person responsible for the change and the date it was made
- Computer-generated or stored data have been identified and that the procedures to protect them against unauthorized amendments or loss are adequate
- The computerized systems used within the study are reliable, accurate and have been validated
- Any unforeseen events recorded in the raw data have been investigated and evaluated
- The results presented in the reports of the study (interim or final) are consistent and complete and that they correctly reflect the raw data

Reporting of Study Results

Purpose: to determine whether final reports are prepared in accordance with GLP principles.

When examining a final report, the inspector should check that:

- It is signed and dated by the study director to indicate acceptance of responsibility for the validity of the study and confirming that the study was conducted in accordance with GLP principles.
- It is signed and dated by other principal scientists, if reports from cooperating disciplines are included.
- A quality assurance statement is included in the report and that it is signed and dated.
- Any amendments were made by the responsible personnel.
- It lists the archive location of all samples, specimens and raw data.

Storage and Retention of Records

Purpose: to determine whether the facility has generated adequate records and reports and whether adequate provision has been made for the safe storage and retention of records and materials.

The inspector should check:

- That a person has been identified as responsible for the archive
- The archive facilities for the storage of study plans, raw data (including that from discontinued GLP studies), final reports, samples and specimens and records of education and training of personnel
- The procedures for retrieval of archived materials
- The procedures whereby access to the archives is limited to authorized personnel and records are kept of personnel given access to raw data, slides, and so on
- That an inventory is maintained of materials removed from, and returned to, the archives
- That records and materials are retained for the required or appropriate period of time and are protected from loss or damage by fire, adverse environmental conditions, and so on

Study Audits

Test facility inspections will generally include, *inter alia*, study audits, which review on-going or completed studies. Specific study audits are also often requested by Regulatory Authorities, and can be conducted independently of test facility inspections. Because of the wide variation in the types of studies which might be audited, only general guidance is appropriate, and inspectors and others taking part in study audits will always need to exercise judgment as to the nature and extent of their examinations. The objective should be to reconstruct the study by comparing the final report with the study plan, relevant SOPs, raw data and other archived material.

In some cases, inspectors may need assistance from other experts in order to conduct an effective study audit, for example, where there is a need to examine tissue sections under the microscope.

When conducting a study audit, the inspector should:

- Obtain names, job descriptions and summaries of training and experience for selected personnel engaged in the study(ies) such as the study director and principal scientists
- Check that there is sufficient staff trained in relevant areas for the study(ies) undertaken
- Identify individual items of apparatus or special equipment used in the study and examine the calibration, maintenance and service records for the equipment
- Review the records relating to the stability of the test substances, analyses of test substance and formulations, analyses of feed, and so on
- Attempt to determine, through the interview process if possible, the work assignments of selected individuals participating in the study to ascertain if these individuals had the time to accomplish the tasks specified in the study plan or report
- Obtain copies of all documentation concerning control procedures or forming integral parts of the study, including:
  - i.   The study plan
  - ii. SOPs in use at the time the study was done
  - iii. Logbooks, laboratory notebooks, files, worksheets, printouts of computer-stored data, and so on; checking of calculations, where appropriate
  - iv. The final report

In studies in which animals (i.e., rodents and other mammals) are used, the inspectors should follow a certain percentage of individual animals from their arrival at the test facility to autopsy. They should pay particular attention to the records relating to:

- Animal body weight, food/water intake, dose formulation and administration, and so on
- Clinical observations and autopsy findings
- Clinical chemistry
- Pathology

Completion of Inspection or Study Audit

When a test facility inspection or study audit has been completed, the inspector should be prepared to discuss his findings with representatives of the test facility at a closing conference and should prepare a written report, that is, the inspection report.

A test facility inspection of any large facility is likely to reveal a number of minor deviations from GLP principles but, normally, these will not be sufficiently serious to affect the validity of studies emanating from that test facility. In such cases, it is reasonable for an inspector to report that the facility is operating in compliance with GLP principles according to the criteria established by the (national) GLP Monitoring Authority. Nevertheless, details of the inadequacies or faults detected should be provided to the test facility and assurances sought from its senior management that action will be taken to remedy them.

The inspector may need to revisit the facility after a period of time to verify that necessary action has been taken.

If a serious deviation from the GLP principles is identified during a test facility inspection or study audit which, in the opinion of the inspector, may have affected the validity of that study, or of other studies performed at the facility, the inspector should report back to the (national) GLP Monitoring Authority. The action taken by that Authority and/or the Regulatory Authority, as appropriate, will depend on the nature and extent of the non-compliance and the legal and/or administrative provisions within the GLP compliance programme.

Where a study audit has been conducted at the request of a Regulatory Authority, a full report of the findings should be prepared and sent via the relevant (national) GLP Monitoring Authority.

ANNEX II
PART A
REPEALED DIRECTIVE AND ITS AMENDMENTS
(Article 9)
>TABLE >
PART B
DEADLINES FOR TRANSPOSITION INTO NATIONAL LAW
(Article 9)
>TABLE >
ANNEX III
CORRELATION TABLE
>TABLE >

QCT-12.4

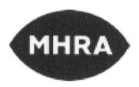

MEDICINES AND HEALTHCARE PRODUCTS REGULATORY AGENCY

STATUTORY INSTRUMENT **1999 No. 3106**

The Good Laboratory Practice Regulations 1999

STATUTORY INSTRUMENTS

1999 No. 3106

HEALTH AND SAFETY

The Good Laboratory Practice Regulations 1999

Made	*18th November 1999*
Laid before Parliament	*19th November 1999*
Coming into force	*14th December 1999*

SCHEDULES

The Secretary of State, being a Minister designated [1] for the purposes of section 2(2) of the European Communities Act 1972 [2] in relation to measures relating to good laboratory practice, in exercise of the powers conferred by the said section 2(2) [3], and of all other powers enabling him in that behalf, hereby makes the following Regulations:

CITATION AND COMMENCEMENT

1. These Regulations may be cited as the Good Laboratory Practice regulations 1999 and shall come into force on 14th December 1999.

INTERPRETATION

2. 1. In these Regulations, unless the context otherwise requires
   "Batch" means a specific quantity or lot of a test or reference item produced during a defined cycle of manufacture in such a way that it could be expected to be of a uniform character;
   "Experimental starting date" means the date on which the first study specific data are collected;
   "Experimental completion date" means the last date on which data are collected from the study;
   "Good laboratory practice instrument" means a document which comprises, or includes
   a. An endorsement by a monitoring authority of a claim by a test facility that the tests that it carries out comply with the principles of good laboratory practice;
   b. A statement by a monitoring authority on the level of adherence of a test facility or a test site to the principles of good laboratory practice (including a statement that the facility or site has been found to be operating in compliance with the said principles or with these Regulations);
   c. A statement by any other person for submission, or which may be submitted, to a regulatory authority on the level of adherence of a test facility or test site, or any part of a test facility or test site, to the principles of good laboratory practice (including a statement that the facility or site operates in compliance with the said principles or with these Regulations);
   d. A statement by any person for submission, or which may be submitted, to a regulatory authority that he is a member of the United Kingdom good laboratory practice compliance programme;
   e. A report issued by a monitoring authority as a result of a study audit or a test facility or test site inspection;
   f. A statement by any person for submission, or which may be submitted, to a regulatory authority about the level of adherence of a regulatory study, or any phase of a regulatory study, to the principles of

good laboratory practice (including a statement that the study, or phase of a study, was conducted in compliance the said principles or with these Regulations), and for the purposes of this definition, the "principles of good laboratory practice" means the said principles howsoever described;

"Master schedule" means a compilation of information to assist in the assessment of workload and for the tracking of studies at a test facility;

"Monitoring authority" means an authority in any country or territory which is responsible (either solely or jointly with other such authorities) for monitoring the good laboratory practice compliance of test facilities;

"OECD" means the Organisation for Economic Cooperation and Development;

"OECD test guideline" means a test guideline which the OECD has recommended for use in its member countries;

"Operator," in relation to a test facility, means the person having control of the test facility;

"Premises," in relation to a test facility, includes field sites at which phases of regulatory studies are conducted;

"Principal investigator" means an individual who, for a multi-site regulatory study, acts on behalf of the study director and has defined responsibility for one or more delegated phases of the study;

"Principles of good laboratory practice" means

a. The principles of good laboratory practice set out in Schedule 1, which are based on the Good Laboratory Practice Principles set out in Section II of the Annex to Council Directive 87/18/ECC[4] on the harmonization of laws, regulations and administrative provisions relating to the application of the principles of good laboratory practice and the verification of their applications for tests on chemical substances, as amended by Commission Directive 1999/11/EC[5] adapting to technical progress the principles of good laboratory practice as specified in Council Directive 87/18/EEC; read with

b. The revised guidance for the conduct of test facility inspections and study audits set out in Schedule 2, which is based on part of the Revised Guidance for the Conduct of Test Facility Inspections and Study Audits in the Annex to Council Directive 88/320/EEC[6] on the inspection and verification of good laboratory practice (GLP), as amended by Commission Directive 1999/12/EC[7] adapting to technical progress for the second time the Annex to Council Directive 88/320/EEC;

"Quality assurance programme" means a defined system, including personnel, which is independent of study conduct and is designed to assure test facility management of compliance with the principles of good laboratory practice;

"Raw data" means all original test facility records and documentation, or verified copies thereof, which are the result of the original observations and activities in a regulatory study;

"Reference item" means any article used to provide a basis for comparison with a test item;

"Regulatory authority" means any authority in any country or territory with legal responsibility for aspects of the control of chemicals or items of natural or biological origin;

"Regulatory study" means a non-clinical experiment or set of experiments

a. In which an item is examined under laboratory conditions or in the environment in order to obtain data on its properties or its safety (or both) with respect to human health, animal health or the environment;
b. The results of which are, or are intended, for submission to the appropriate regulatory authorities; and
c. Compliance with the principles of good laboratory practice is required in respect of that experiment or set of experiments by the appropriate regulatory authorities (whether or not compliance with the said principles in respect of that experiment or set of experiments is also a legislative requirement);

"Short-term study" means a regulatory study of short duration with widely used, routine techniques;

"Specimen" means any material derived from a test system for examination, analysis, or retention;

"Sponsor" means a person who commissions, supports and/or submits a regulatory study;

"Standard operating procedures" means the documented procedures which describe how to perform tests or activities normally not specified in detail in study plans or test guidelines;

"Study completion date" means the date the study director signs the final report;

"Study director" means the individual responsible for the overall conduct of the regulatory study;

"Study initiation date" means the date the study director (first) signs the study plan;

"Study plan" means a document which defines the objectives and experimental design for the conduct of a regulatory study, and includes any study plan amendments;

"Study plan amendment" means an intended change to the study plan after the study initiation date;

"Study plan deviation" means an unintended departure from the study plan after the study initiation date;

"Test facility" means a facility which conducts or intends to conduct regulatory studies;

"Test item" means an article that is the subject of a regulatory study;

"Test site" means a location at which a phase of a regulatory study is conducted;

"Test system" means any biological, chemical or physical system or a combination thereof used in a regulatory study;

"Vehicle" means any agent which serves as a carrier used to mix, disperse, or solubilize the test or reference item to facilitate the administration or application to the test system.

2. In these Regulations, unless the context otherwise requires, a reference

    a. To a numbered regulation or Schedule is to the regulation in or Schedule to these Regulations bearing that number;

    b. In a regulation to a numbered or lettered paragraph is to the paragraph of that regulation bearing that number or letter; and

    c. In a paragraph to a numbered or lettered sub-paragraph is to the sub-paragraph in that paragraph bearing that number or letter.

THE GOOD LABORATORY PRACTICE MONITORING AUTHORITY

3. 1. The body responsible for enforcing compliance with these Regulations shall be the Good Laboratory Practice Monitoring Authority, a body consisting of the Secretary of State for Health, the National Assembly for Wales, the Scottish Ministers and the Department of Health and Social Services for Northern Ireland.

    2. The functions of the Good Laboratory Practice Monitoring Authority may be performed by any one of the Secretary of State for Health, the National Assembly for Wales, the Scottish Ministers or the Department of Health and Social Services for Northern Ireland acting alone, or any two or more of them acting jointly.

    3. In accordance with the preceding provisions of this regulation, in these Regulations, "the Good Laboratory Practice Monitoring Authority" ("the GLPMA") means any one or more of the Secretary of State for Health, the National Assembly for Wales, the Scottish Ministers and the Department of Health and Social Services for Northern Ireland, and, in the case of anything falling to be done by the GLPMA, means any one or more of them acting as mentioned in paragraph (2).

    4. The GLPMA may appoint such persons as they think necessary for the proper discharge by them of their functions, and those persons shall be appointed upon such terms and conditions (including conditions as to remuneration, benefits, allowances and reimbursement for expenses) as the GLPMA think fit.

REQUIREMENT TO BE A MEMBER OR A PROSPECTIVE MEMBER OF THE UNITED KINGDOM GOOD LABORATORY PRACTICE COMPLIANCE PROGRAMME

4. A regulatory study shall not be conducted at any premises of a test facility unless

a. The operator of the test facility is regarded by virtue of regulation 5 or 6 as a member or a prospective member of the United Kingdom good laboratory practice compliance programme (hereafter referred to as "the UK GLP compliance programme"); and

b. The operator's membership or prospective membership of that programme is or is partly in respect of those premises,

and if a regulatory study is conducted at any premises in contravention of this regulation, the operator of that test facility shall be guilty of an offence.

PROSPECTIVE MEMBERSHIP OF THE UNITED KINGDOM GOOD LABORATORY PRACTICE COMPLIANCE PROGRAMME

5. 1. An operator of a test facility shall, for the purposes of these Regulations, be regarded as being a prospective member of the UK GLP compliance programme in respect of particular premises only if -

a. He has informed the GLPMA by notice in writing of the intention to conduct regulatory studies at those premises;

b. The GLPMA has in writing -

   i. Acknowledged receipt of that notification, and

   ii. Informed the operator that he is a prospective member of the programme in respect of those premises,

and he has not ceased to be regarded as a prospective member of the programme in respect of those premises by virtue of paragraph (2).

2. An operator of a test facility shall cease to be regarded as a prospective member of the UK GLP compliance programme in respect of particular test facility premises if

a. He is admitted to membership of the programme in respect of those premises by the GLPMA;

b. He informs the GLPMA in writing that he no longer conducts or intends to conduct regulatory studies at those premises; or

c. Subject to paragraph (3), the GLPMA inform him in writing that they are not prepared to admit him to membership of the programme in respect of those premises.

3. The GLPMA shall, before informing a prospective member of the UK GLP compliance programme they are not prepared to admit him to membership of the programme in respect of particular test facility premises:

a. Inform the prospective member that they are considering taking such action and explain to him in writing the reasons why such action is being considered;

b. Give the operator a specified period within which to make representations to the GLPMA; and

c. Consider any representations which are duly made and not withdrawn, unless, for either of the reasons set out in paragraph (4), it is necessary for the GLPMA to inform the prospective member immediately that they are not prepared to admit him to membership of the programme in respect of those premises.

4. The reasons referred to in paragraph (3) are that
   a. There is a failure to adhere to the principles of good laboratory practice at those premises which, in the opinion of the GLPMA, may contribute towards precipitating a danger to animal or human health or to the environment; or
   b. To ensure fulfilment of a Community obligation.

MEMBERSHIP OF THE UNITED KINGDOM GOOD LABORATORY PRACTICE COMPLIANCE PROGRAMME

6. 1. Subject to paragraph (2) and except where paragraph (5), (6) or (7) applies, the operator of a test facility shall be regarded as being a member of the UK GLP compliance programme in respect of particular test facility premises if
   a. He was regarded as being a member of the programme in respect of those premises immediately before these Regulations come into force by virtue of regulation 6 of the Good Laboratory Practice Regulations 1997 [8]; or
   b. After having inspected those premises, the GLPMA have informed the operator in writing that they are admitting the operator to membership of the programme in respect of those premises.

2. The operator of a test facility shall cease to be a member of the UK GLP compliance programme in respect of particular test facility premises if
   a. He has informed the GLPMA in writing that regulatory studies are no longer conducted at those premises; or
   b. Membership of the programme in respect of those premises has been withdrawn by the GLPMA in accordance with paragraph (3).

3. Subject to paragraph (4), the GLPMA may by a notice in writing served on the operator of a test facility withdraw the operator's membership of the UK GLP compliance programme in respect of particular test facility premises if
   a. The operator, in the opinion of the GLPMA, no longer intends to conduct regulatory studies at those premises;
   b. The operator is, in the opinion of the GLPMA, not capable of ensuring that the principles of good laboratory practice are adhered to at those premises; or
   c. At those premises there is a failure to adhere to the principles of good laboratory practice which, in the opinion of the GLPMA, may contribute towards precipitating a danger to animal or human health or to the environment.

4. Before serving a notice on an operator of a test facility under paragraph (3) (a) or (b), the GLPMA shall -
   a. inform the operator in writing that they are considering serving such a notice and explain to him in writing the reasons why they are considering serving such a notice;

b. give the operator a specified period within which to make representations to him; and

c. consider any representations which are duly made and not withdrawn, unless, in order to ensure fulfilment of any Community obligation, it is necessary for the GLPMA to serve the notice immediately.

5. Where an operator of a test facility has ceased to be a member of the UK GLP compliance programme in respect of particular test facility premises on the grounds set out in paragraph (2)(a), or membership of the programme in respect of particular test facility premises has been withdrawn from him on the grounds set out in paragraph (3)(a), he shall again be regarded as being a member of the programme in respect of those premises if -

a. he has informed the GLPMA by notice in writing of the intention to conduct further regulatory studies at those premises;

b. he has become a prospective member of the programme in respect of those premises in accordance with the procedure set out in regulation 5; and

c. after having inspected those premises, the GLPMA has informed the operator in writing of his readmission to membership of the programme in respect of those premises.

6. Where membership of the UK GLP compliance programme has been withdrawn from an operator of a test facility in respect of particular test facility premises on the grounds set out in paragraph (3)(b), he shall again be regarded as being a member of the programme in respect of those premises if -

a. he has informed the GLPMA by notice in writing of the intention to conduct further regulatory studies at those premises; and

b. the GLPMA -

   i. are of the opinion that the operator is capable of ensuring that the principles of good laboratory practice are adhered to at those premises, and

   ii. have informed the operator in writing of his readmission to membership of the programme in respect of those premises.

7. Where membership of the UK GLP compliance programme has been withdrawn from an operator of a test facility in respect of particular test facility premises on the grounds set out in paragraph (3)(c), he shall again be regarded as being a member of the programme in respect of those premises if -

a. he has informed the GLPMA by notice in writing of the intention to conduct further regulatory studies at those premises; and

b. the GLPMA -

   i. are of the opinion that the possible danger to animal or human health or to the environment which led to membership being withdrawn is no longer present, and

   ii. have informed the operator in writing of his readmission to membership of the programme in respect of those premises.

Requirement to Adhere to the Principles of Good Laboratory Practice

7. 1. No person shall conduct a regulatory study at any premises of a test facility unless with regard to that study the principles of good laboratory practice are adhered to -
   a. as respects the organizational structure surrounding the study; and
   b. as respects the conditions under which the study is planned, performed, monitored, recorded, archived and reported.

2. If the GLPMA have reasonable grounds for believing that a person has contravened paragraph (1) and is responsible for a serious deviation from the principles of good laboratory practice which may have affected the validity of a regulatory study, they may by a notice served on the operator of the test facility at whose premises the alleged contravention took place (in these Regulations referred to as a "warning notice") -
   a. state the GLPMA's grounds for believing that the person -
      i. has contravened paragraph (1), and
      ii. is responsible for a serious deviation from the principles of good laboratory practice which may have affected the validity of a regulatory study;
   b. specify the measures which, in the opinion of the GLPMA, the operator of the test facility must take in order to ensure that the serious deviation from the principles of good laboratory practice which may have affected the validity of a regulatory study will not recur;
   c. require the operator of the test facility to take those measures, or measures which are at least equivalent to them, within such period as may be specified in the warning notice; and
   d. inform the operator of the test facility of -
      i. his right of appeal against the warning notice under regulation 8,
      ii. the period within which such an appeal may be brought, and
      iii. the effect that such an appeal will have on any criminal proceedings relating to the operator's alleged failure to comply with the warning notice.

3. Any operator of a test facility who fails to comply with a warning notice shall, unless that notice has been withdrawn by the GLPMA or cancelled by a court, be guilty of an offence.

Appeals against Warning Notices

8. 1. An operator of a test facility who is aggrieved by a decision to serve a warning notice on him may appeal -
   a. in England, Wales or Northern Ireland, to a magistrates' court, and such an appeal shall be by way of complaint for an order; or
   b. in Scotland, to a sheriff, and such an appeal shall be by summary application.

2. The period during which such an appeal may be brought is -
   a. one month from the date on which the warning notice was served on the operator desiring to appeal; or
   b. the period specified in the warning notice,
   whichever ends the earlier.
3. On an appeal against a warning notice, a magistrates' or sheriff court may either cancel or affirm the notice and, if it affirms it, may do so either in its original form or with such modifications as the court may, in the circumstances, think fit.
4. Pending the final disposal of an appeal, unless or until the appeal is withdrawn, any criminal proceedings relating the operator's alleged failure to comply with the warning notice shall be stayed or suspended.

Powers of Entry and so on

9. 1. For the purposes of enforcing compliance with these Regulations, a person appointed in accordance with regulation 3(4) shall have a right -
   a. at any reasonable hour to enter any premises other than premises used only as a private dwelling house which he has reason to believe it is necessary for him to visit;
   b. to carry out at those premises during that visit such inspections, examinations, tests and analyses as he considers necessary;
   c. to require the production of and inspect any article or substances at the premises;
   d. to require the production of, inspect and take copies of or extracts from any book, document, data or record (in whatever form it is held) at, or (in the case of computer data or records) accessible at, the premises;
   e. subject to paragraph (5), to take possession of any article, substance, book, document, data, record (in whatever form they are held) at, or (in the case of computer data or records) accessible at, the premises;
   f. to question any person whom he finds at the premises and whom he has reasonable cause to believe is able to give him relevant information;
   g. to require any person to afford him such assistance as he considers necessary with respect to any matter within that person's control or in relation to which that person has responsibilities;
   h. to require, as he considers necessary, any person to afford him such facilities as he may reasonably require that person to afford him,
   but nothing in this paragraph shall be taken to compel the production by any person of a document of which he would, on grounds of legal professional privilege, be entitled to withhold production on an order for disclosure in an action in the High Court or, as the case may be, on an order for the production of documents in an action in the Court of Session.
2. If a justice of the peace is satisfied by any written information on oath that there are reasonable grounds for entry into any premises other than premises

used only as a private dwelling house for any purpose mentioned in paragraph (1), and -

a. admission to the premises has been or is likely to be refused and notice of intention to apply for a warrant under this subsection has been given to the occupier; or

b. an application for admission, or the giving of such notice, would defeat the object of the entry or that the premises are unoccupied or that the occupier is temporarily absent and it might defeat the object of the entry to await his return,

the justice may be by warrant signed by him, which shall continue in force for a period of one month, authorize any person appointed in accordance with regulation 3(4) to enter the premises, if need be by force.

3. A person appointed in accordance with regulation 3(4) entering any premises by virtue of paragraph (1) or of a warrant under paragraph (2) may take with him when he enters those premises such equipment as may appear to him necessary and any person who is authorized by the GLPMA to accompany him on that visit.

4. On leaving any premises which a person appointed in accordance with regulation 3(4) is authorized to enter by a warrant under paragraph (2), that person shall, if the premises are unoccupied or the occupier is temporarily absent, leave the premises as effectively secured against trespassers as he found them.

5. Where, pursuant to paragraph (1)(e), a person appointed in accordance with regulation 3(4) takes possession of any article, substance, book, document, data or record, he shall leave at the premises with a responsible person a statement giving particulars of the article, substance, book, document, data or record sufficient to identify it and stating that he has taken possession of it.

6. Persons appointed in accordance with regulation 3(4) shall, when enforcing compliance with these Regulations, have regard to any relevant provision of the Revised Guidance for the Conduct of Test Facility Inspections and Study Audits set out in Part B of the Annex to Council Directive 88/320/EEC on the inspection and verification of good laboratory practice (GLP), as amended by Commission Directive 1999/12/EC adapting to technical progress for the second time the Annex to Council Directive 88/320/EEC.

DISCLOSURE OF CONFIDENTIAL INFORMATION

10. 1. A person who in the course of enforcing compliance with these Regulations gains access to commercially sensitive or other confidential information shall be guilty of an offence if, without lawful authority, he discloses that information.

2. A person may disclose commercially sensitive or other confidential information to which he has had access in the course of enforcing compliance with these Regulations to -

    a. the European Commission;

    b. a monitoring authority;

    c. a regulatory authority;

    d. a police force;

    e. a test facility or sponsor concerned with the inspection or study audit during the course of which the GLPMA gained access to that information.

  3. For the purposes of this regulation -

    a. the names of test facilities or test sites which are or have been subject to an inspection as part of the UK GLP compliance programme;

    b. the level of adherence of a test facility or test site to the principles of good laboratory practice of those laboratories as assessed by the GLPMA; and

    c. the dates upon which study audits or test facility or test site inspections have been conducted,

  shall not be considered to be confidential.

OBSTRUCTION AND SO ON OF AUTHORISED PERSONS

11. 1. Subject to paragraph (2) -

    a. any person who -

      i. intentionally obstructs a person appointed in accordance with regulation 3(4), or

      ii. without reasonable cause fails to comply with any requirement made of him by a person appointed in accordance with regulation 3(4),

    in circumstances where that person is acting in pursuance of any of his functions under these Regulations; or

    b. any person who, in purported compliance with any such requirement as is mentioned in sub-paragraph (a)(ii), intentionally or recklessly furnishes information which is false or misleading in a material particular,

    shall be guilty of an offence.

  2. Nothing in paragraph (1)(a)(ii) shall be construed as requiring any person to answer any question or give any information if to do so might incriminate him or, in the case of a person who is married, his spouse.

FALSE GOOD LABORATORY PRACTICE INSTRUMENTS

12. 1. A person who

    a. makes a false good laboratory practice instrument; or

    b. makes a copy of an instrument which is, and which he knows or believes to be, a false good laboratory practice instrument,

  with the intention that he or another shall use it to induce a regulatory authority to accept it as a genuine good laboratory practice instrument or a copy of a genuine good laboratory practice instrument shall be guilty of an offence.

2. A person who has in his possession
   a. a false good laboratory practice instrument which he knows or believes to be a false good laboratory practice instrument;
   b. a copy of an instrument which he knows or believes to be a false good laboratory practice instrument,

   with the intention that he or another shall supply it to a regulatory authority with the intention of inducing the regulatory authority to accept it as a genuine good laboratory practice instrument or a copy of a genuine good laboratory practice instrument shall be guilty of an offence.
3. A person who supplies to a regulatory authority
   a. a false good laboratory practice instrument which he knows or believes to be a false good laboratory practice instrument;
   b. a copy of an instrument which he knows or believes to be a false good laboratory practice instrument,

   with the intention of inducing the regulatory authority to accept it as a genuine good laboratory practice instrument or a copy of a genuine good laboratory practice instrument shall be guilty of an offence.
4. A good laboratory practice instrument is "false" for the purposes of this regulation if
   a. it is not that which it purports to be for any reason including where -
      i. it purports to have been made by a person who did not make it,
      ii. it purports to have been made in the form in which it is made by a person who did not in fact make it in that form,
      iii. it purports to have been altered in any respect on the authority of a person who did not in fact authorize the alteration in that respect; or
   b. it includes information which is false or misleading in a material particular,

   and a person shall be treated for the purposes of this regulation as making a false good laboratory practice instrument if he alters a good laboratory practice instrument so as to make it false in any respect (whether or not it is false in some other respect apart from that alteration).
5. A person may be guilty of an offence
   a. under paragraph (1) or (2) if the regulatory authority is outside the United Kingdom;
   b. under paragraph (3) if the supply is from outside the United Kingdom to a United Kingdom regulatory authority or from within the United Kingdom to a regulatory authority outside the United Kingdom.

OFFENCES BY BODIES CORPORATE AND SCOTTISH PARTNERSHIPS

13. Where an offence under these Regulations is committed by a body corporate or Scottish partnership and is proved to have been committed with the consent or connivance of, or to be attributable to any neglect on the part of -

a. any director, manager, secretary, partner or similar officer of the body corporate or Scottish partnership; or
b. any person who was purporting to act in any such capacity,
   he as well as the body corporate or Scottish partnership shall be deemed to be guilty of that offence and he shall be liable to be proceeded against and punished accordingly.

DEFENCE OF DUE DILIGENCE

14. In any proceedings for an offence under any of the preceding provisions of these Regulations, it shall be a defence for the person charged to prove that he took all reasonable precautions and exercised all due diligence to avoid the commission of the offence.

PENALTIES

15. A person guilty of
   a. an offence under regulation 11(1)(a) shall be liable on summary conviction to a fine not exceeding level 3 on the standard scale;
   b. an offence under regulation 12 shall be liable
      i. on summary conviction to a fine not exceeding the statutory maximum or to imprisonment for a term not exceeding three months or to both,
      ii. on conviction on indictment to a fine or to imprisonment for a term not exceeding two years or to both;
   c. any other offence under these Regulations shall be liable on summary conviction to a fine not exceeding level 5 on the standard scale or to imprisonment for a term not exceeding three months or both.

FEES

16. 1. The GLPMA may charge operators of test facilities and operators of test facilities shall, if so charged, pay to the GLPMA such reasonable fees as the GLPMA may determine to cover the cost of providing inspections and services under these Regulations.
   2. The GLPMA may set those fees at levels such that they meet that part of the expenditure of the GLPMA which is reasonably attributable to the cost of inspecting and providing services under these Regulations to or on behalf of the person or class of person charged but the fees must not include any element of profit.
   3. Any such fee shall be payable within fourteen days following written notice from the GLPMA requiring payment of the fee.
   4. All unpaid sums due by way of, or on account of, any fees payable under this regulation shall be recoverable as debts due to the Crown.

5. The GLPMA may in exceptional circumstances
   a. waive payment of any fee or reduce any fee or part of a fee otherwise payable under this regulation;
   b. refund the whole or part of any fee paid pursuant to this regulation.

REVOCATION

17. The Good Laboratory Practice Regulations 1997 are hereby revoked.

Alan Milburn

One of Her Majesty's Principal Secretaries of State

Department of Health
18th November 1999

SCHEDULE 1

Regulation 2(1)

GOOD LABORATORY PRACTICE PRINCIPLES (BASED ON SECTION II OF THE ANNEX TO COUNCIL DIRECTIVE 87/18/EEC, AS AMENDED BY COMMISSION DIRECTIVE 1999/11/EC)

PART I

TEST FACILITY ORGANISATION AND PERSONNEL

FACILITY MANAGEMENT'S RESPONSIBILITIES

1. 1. Each test facility management should ensure that the principles of good laboratory practice are complied with in its test facility.
   2. As a minimum it should -
   a. ensure that a statement exists which identifies the individuals within a test facility who fulfill the responsibilities of management as defined by the principles of good laboratory practice;
   b. ensure that a sufficient number of qualified personnel, appropriate facilities, equipment, and materials are available for the timely and proper conduct or regulatory studies;
   c. ensure the maintenance of a record of the qualifications, training, experience and job description for each professional and technical individual;
   d. ensure that personnel clearly understand the functions they are to perform and, where necessary, provide training for those functions;

   e. ensure that appropriate and technically valid standard operating procedures are established and followed, and approve all original and revised standard operating procedures;

   f. ensure that there is a quality assurance programme with designated personnel and assure that the quality assurance programme is being performed in accordance with the principles of good laboratory practice;

   g. ensure that for each study an individual with the appropriate qualifications, training and experience is designated by the management as the study director before the study is initiated. Replacement of a study director should be done according to established procedures, and should be documented;

   h. ensure, in the event of a multi-site study, that, if needed, a principal investigator is designated, who is appropriately trained, qualified and experienced to supervise any delegated phase of the study. Replacement of the principal investigator should be done according to established procedures, and should be documented;

   i. ensure documented approval of the study plan by the study director;

   j. ensure that the study director has made the approved study plan available to the quality assurance personnel;

   k. ensure maintenance of a historical file of all standard operating procedures;

   l. ensure that an individual is identified as responsible for the management of the archives;

   m. ensure maintenance of a master schedule;

   n. ensure that test facility supplies meet requirements appropriate to their use in a study;

   o. ensure for a multi-site study that clear lines of communication exist between the study director, principal investigator, quality assurance programme and personnel;

   p. ensure that test and reference items are appropriately characterized;

   q. establish procedures to ensure that computerized systems are suitable for their intended purpose, and are validated, operated and maintained in accordance with the principles of good laboratory practice.

3. When a phase of a study is conducted at a test site, test site management (if appointed) will have the responsibilities set out in sub-paragraph (2)(a) to (f), (h), (k) to (n), (p) and (q).

STUDY DIRECTOR'S RESPONSIBILITIES

2. 1. The study director is the single point of study control and has the responsibility for the overall conduct of the regulatory study and for its final report.

   2. These responsibilities should include, but not be limited to, the following functions. The study director should

a. approve the study plan and any amendments to the study plan by dated signature;
b. ensure that the quality assurance personnel have a copy of the study plan and any amendments in a timely manner and communicate effectively with the quality assurance personnel as required during the conduct of the study;
c. ensure that study plans and amendments and standard operating procedures are available to study personnel;
d. ensure that the study plan and the final report for a multi-site study identify and define the role of any principal investigators and any test facilities and test sites involved in the conduct of the study;
e. ensure that the procedures specified in the study plan are followed, and assess and document the impact of any deviations from the study plan on the quality and integrity of the study, and take appropriate corrective action if necessary; and acknowledge deviations from standard operating procedures during the conduct of the study;
f. ensure that all raw data generated are fully documented and recorded;
g. ensure that computerized systems used in the study have been validated;
h. sign and date the final report to indicate acceptance of responsibility for the validity of the data and to indicate the extent to which the study complies with the principles of good laboratory practice;
i. ensure that after completion (including termination) of the regulatory study, the study plan, the final report, raw data and supporting material are archived.

PRINCIPAL INVESTIGATOR'S RESPONSIBILITIES

3. The principal investigator will ensure that the delegated phases of the study are conducted in accordance with the applicable principles of good laboratory practice.

STUDY PERSONNEL'S RESPONSIBILITIES

4. 1. All personnel involved in the conduct of the regulatory study must be knowledgeable in those parts of the principles of good laboratory practice which are applicable to their involvement in the study.
2. Study personnel will have access to the regulatory study plan and appropriate standard operating procedures applicable to their involvement in the study. It is their responsibility to comply with the instructions given in these documents. Any deviation from these instructions should be documented and communicated directly to the study director and/or, if appropriate, the principal investigator.

3. All study personnel are responsible for recording raw data promptly and accurately and in compliance with these principles of good laboratory practice, and are responsible for the quality of their data.

4. Study personnel should exercise health precautions to minimize risk to themselves and to ensure the integrity of the regulatory study. They should communicate to the appropriate person any relevant known health or medical condition in order that they can be excluded from operations that may affect the study.

PART II

QUALITY ASSURANCE PROGRAMME

GENERAL

1. 1. The test facility should have a documented quality assurance programme to assure that regulatory studies performed are in compliance with the principles of good laboratory practice.

2. The quality assurance programme should be carried out by an individual or by individuals designated by and directly responsible to management and who are familiar with the test procedures.

3. This individual or these individuals should not be involved in the conduct of the regulatory study being assured.

RESPONSIBILITIES OF THE QUALITY ASSURANCE PERSONNEL

2. The responsibilities of the quality assurance personnel should include, but not be limited to, the following functions. They should

   a. maintain copies of all approved study plans and standard operating procedures in use in the test facility and have access to an up-to-date copy of the master schedule;

   b. verify that the study plan contains the information required for compliance with the principles of good laboratory practice. The verification should be documented;

   c. conduct inspections to determine if all studies are conducted in accordance with the principles of good laboratory practice. Inspections should also determine that study plans and standard operating procedures have been made available to study personnel and are being followed. Inspections can be of three types, as specified by quality assurance programme standard operating procedures
      - study based inspections,
      - facility based inspections,
      - process based inspections,
      and records of such inspections should be retained;

   d. inspect the final reports to confirm that the methods, procedures, and observations are accurately and completely described, and that the reported results accurately and completely reflect the raw data of the regulatory study;

e. promptly report any inspection results in writing to management and to the study director, and to any principal investigator and the respective management, when applicable;

f. prepare and sign a statement, to be included with the final report, which specifies the types of inspections and their dates, including the phase of a study inspected, and the dates inspection results were reported to management and the study director and any principal investigators, if applicable. This statement would also serve to confirm that the final report reflects the raw data.

PART III

FACILITIES

GENERAL

1. 1. The test facility should be of suitable size, construction and location to meet the requirements of the regulatory study and to minimize disturbance that would interfere with the validity of the regulatory study.

  2. The design of the test facility should provide an adequate degree of separation of the different activities to assure the proper conduct of each regulatory study.

TEST SYSTEM FACILITIES

2. 1. The test facility should have a sufficient number of rooms or areas to assure the isolation of test systems and the isolation of individual projects, involving substances known or suspected of being biohazardous.

  2. Suitable facilities should be available for the diagnosis, treatment and control of diseases, in order to ensure that there is no unacceptable degree of deterioration of test systems.

  3. There should be storage rooms or areas as needed for supplies and equipment. Storage rooms or areas should be separated from rooms or areas housing the test systems and should provide adequate protection against infestation, contamination and deterioration.

FACILITIES FOR HANDLING TEST AND REFERENCE ITEMS

3. 1. To prevent contamination or mix-ups, there should be separate rooms or areas for receipt and storage of the test and reference items, and mixing of the test items with a vehicle.

  2. Storage rooms or areas for the test items should be separate from rooms or areas containing the test systems. They should be adequate to preserve identity, concentration, purity and stability, and ensure safe storage for hazardous substances.

ARCHIVE FACILITIES

4. Archive facilities should be provided for the secure storage and retrieval of study plans, raw data, final reports, samples of test items and specimens. Archive design and archive conditions should protect contents from untimely deterioration.

WASTE DISPOSAL

5. Handling and disposal of wastes should be carried out in such a way as not to jeopardize the integrity of regulatory studies. This includes provision for appropriate collection, storage and disposal facilities, and decontamination and transportation procedures.

PART IV

APPARATUS, MATERIALS AND REAGENTS

1. Apparatus, including validated computerized systems, used for the generation, storage and retrieval of data, and for controlling environmental factors relevant to the regulatory study, should be suitably located and of appropriate design and adequate capacity.

2. Apparatus used in a regulatory study should be periodically inspected, cleaned, maintained, and calibrated according to standard operating procedures. Records of these activities should be maintained. Calibration should, where appropriate, be traceable to national or international standards of measurement.

3. Apparatus and materials used in studies should not interfere adversely with the test systems.

4. Chemicals, reagents and solutions should be labelled to indicate identity (with concentration if appropriate), expiry date and specific storage instructions. Information concerning source, preparation date and stability should be available. The expiry date may be extended on the basis of documented evaluation or analysis.

PART V

TEST SYSTEMS

PHYSICAL/CHEMICAL

1. 1. Apparatus used for the generation of physical/chemical data should be suitably located and of appropriate design and adequate capacity.
   2. The integrity of the physical/chemical test systems should be ensured.

BIOLOGICAL

2. 1. Proper conditions should be established and maintained for the storage, housing, handling and care of biological test systems, in order to ensure the quality of the data.

2. Newly received animal and plant test systems should be isolated until their health status has been evaluated. If any unusual mortality or morbidity occurs, the relevant lot should not be used in regulatory studies and, where appropriate, should be humanely destroyed. At the experimental starting date of a regulatory study, test systems should be free of any disease or condition that might interfere with the purpose or conduct of the study. Test systems that become diseased or injured during the course of a regulatory study should be isolated and treated, if necessary to maintain the integrity of the study. Any diagnosis and treatment of any disease before or during a regulatory study should be recorded.

3. Records of source, date of arrival and the arrival condition of test systems should be maintained.

4. Biological test systems should be acclimatized to the test environment for an adequate period before the first administration or application of the test or reference item.

5. All information needed to identify properly the test systems should appear on their housing or containers. Individual test systems that are to be removed from their housing or containers during the conduct of the regulatory study should bear appropriate identification, wherever possible.

6. During use, housing or containers for test systems should be cleaned and sanitized at appropriate intervals. Any material that comes into contact with the test system should be free of contaminants at levels that would interfere with the regulatory study. Bedding for animals should be changed as required by sound husbandry practice. Use of pest control agents should be documented.

7. Test systems used in field studies should be located so as to avoid interference in the regulatory study from spray drift and from past usage of pesticides.

PART VI

TEST AND REFERENCE ITEMS

RECEIPT, HANDLING, SAMPLING AND STORAGE

1. 1. Records including test item and reference item characterization, date of receipt, expiry date, quantities received and used in regulatory studies should be maintained.

2. Handling, sampling and storage procedures should be identified in order that the homogeneity and stability are assured to the degree possible and contamination or mix-up are precluded.
3. Storage containers should carry identification information, expiry date and specific storage instructions.

CHARACTERIZATION

2. 1. Each test and reference item should be appropriately identified (eg code, chemical abstracts service registry number (CAS number), name, biological parameters etc.).
2. For each regulatory study, the identity, including batch number, purity, composition, concentrations or other characteristics to appropriately define each batch of the test or reference items should be known.
3. In cases where the test item is supplied by the sponsor, there should be a mechanism, developed in co-operation between the sponsor and the test facility, to verify the identity of the test item subject to the study.
4. The stability of test and reference items under storage and test conditions should be known for all regulatory studies.
5. If the test item is administered or applied in a vehicle, the homogeneity, concentration and stability of the test item in that vehicle should be determined. For test items used in field studies (eg tank mixes), these may be determined through separate laboratory experiments.
6. A sample for analytical purposes from each batch of test item should be retained for all regulatory studies except short-term studies.

PART VII

STANDARD OPERATING PROCEDURES

1. A test facility should have written standard operating procedures approved by test facility management that are intended to ensure the quality and integrity of the data generated by the test facility. Revisions to standard operating procedures should be approved by test facility management.
2. Each separate test facility unit or area should have immediately available current standard operating procedures relevant to the activities being performed therein. Published textbooks, analytical methods, articles and manuals may be used as supplements to these standard operating procedures.
3. Deviations from standard operating procedures related to the regulatory study should be documented and should be acknowledged by the study director and any principal investigators, as applicable.

4. Standard operating procedures should be available for, but not be limited to, the following categories of test facility activities. The details given under each heading are to be considered as illustrative examples -

a. **Test and reference items**
   receipt, identification, labelling, handling, sampling and storage

b. **Apparatus, materials and reagents**
   i. *apparatus:* use, maintenance, cleaning and calibration
   ii. *computerized systems:* validation, operation, maintenance, security, change control and back-up
   iii. *materials, reagents and solutions:* preparation and labelling

c. **Record keeping, reporting, storage, and retrieval**
   coding of studies, data collection, preparation of reports, indexing systems, handling of data, including the use of computerized data systems

d. **Test system (where appropriate)**
   i. room preparation and environmental room conditions for the test system
   ii. procedures for receipt, transfer, proper placement, characterization, identification and care of test system
   iii. test system preparation, observation and examinations, before, during and at the conclusion of the regulatory study
   iv. handling of test system individuals found moribund or dead during the regulatory study
   v. collection, identification and handling of specimens including necropsy and histopathology
   vi. siting and placement of test systems in test plots

e. **Quality assurance procedures**
   operation of quality assurance personnel in planning, scheduling, performing, documenting and reporting inspections

PART VIII

PERFORMANCE OF THE REGULATORY STUDY

STUDY PLAN

1. 1. For each regulatory study, a written plan should exist prior to initiation of the study. The study plan should be approved by dated signature of the study director and verified for good laboratory practice compliance by quality assurance personnel as specified in paragraph 2(b) of Part II of this Schedule.

2. As respects the study plan -
   a. amendments to it should be justified and approved by dated signature
      of the study director and maintained with the study plan;
   b. deviations from it should be described, explained, acknowledged and
      dated in a timely fashion by the study director and/or any principal
      investigators and maintained with the study raw data.
3. For short-term studies, a general study plan accompanied by a study specific
   supplement may be used.

CONTENT OF THE STUDY PLAN

2. 1. The study plan should contain, but not be limited to, the following
   information
   a. **Identification of the study, the test item and the reference item**
      i.   a descriptive title
      ii. a statement which reveals the nature and purpose of the regulatory
           study
      iii. identification of the test item by code or name (IUPAC, CAS num-
           ber, biological parameters, etc.)
      iv. the reference item to be used
   b. **Information concerning the sponsor and the test facility**
      i.   name and address of the sponsor
      ii. name and address of any test facilities and test sites involved
      iii. name and address of the study director
      iv. name and address of any principal investigator, and the phase of the
           study delegated by the study director to, and under the responsibility
           of, the principal investigator
   c. **Dates**
      i.   the date of approval of the study plan by signature of the study
           director
      ii. the proposed experimental starting and completion dates
   d. **Test methods**
      reference to OECD test guideline or other test guideline or method to
      be used
   e. **Issues (where applicable)**
      i.   the justification for selection of the test system
      ii. characterization of the test system, such as the species, strain, sub-
           strain, source of supply, number, body weight range, sex, age, and
           other pertinent information
      iii. the method of administration and the reason for its choice
      iv. the dose levels and/or concentration, frequency, duration of admin-
           istration or application
      v.   detailed information on the experimental design, including a des-
           cription of the chronological procedure of the regulatory study, all
           methods, materials and conditions, type and frequency of analysis,

measurements, observations and examinations to be performed, and statistical methods to be used (if any)

f. **Records**
a list of records to be retained

CONDUCT OF THE REGULATORY STUDY

3. 1. a unique identification should be given to each regulatory study. All items concerning this regulatory study should carry this identification. Specimens from the study should be identified to confirm their origin. Such identification should enable traceability, as appropriate for the specimen and study.

2. The regulatory study should be conducted in accordance with the study plan.

3. All data generated during the conduct of the regulatory study should be recorded directly, promptly, accurately and legibly by the individual entering the data. These entries should be signed or initialled and dated.

4. Any change in the raw data should be made so as not to obscure the previous entry, should indicate the reason for change and should be dated and signed or initialled by the individual making the change.

5. Data generated as a direct computer input should be identified at the time of data input by the individual responsible for direct data entries. Computerized system design should always provide for the retention of full audit trails to show all changes to the data without obscuring the original data. It should be possible to associate all changes to data with the person having made those changes, for example by the use of timed and dated (electronic) signatures. Reasons for changes should be given.

PART IX

REPORTING OF REGULATORY STUDY RESULTS

GENERAL

1. 1. A final report should be prepared for each regulatory study. In the case of short-term studies, a standardized final report accompanied by a study specific extension may be prepared.

2. Reports of principal investigators or scientists involved in the regulatory study should be signed and dated by them.

3. The final report should be signed and dated by the study director to indicate acceptance of responsibility for the validity of the data. The extent of compliance with these principles of good laboratory practice should be indicated.

4. Corrections and additions to a final report should be in the form of amendments. Amendments should clearly specify the reason for the corrections or additions and should be signed and dated by the study director.

5. Reformatting of the final report to comply with the submission requirements of a national registration or regulatory authority does not constitute a correction, addition or amendment to the final report.

CONTENT OF THE FINAL REPORT

2. The final report should include, but not be limited to, the following information -

    a. **Identification of the regulatory study, the test item and the reference item**
       i. a descriptive title
      ii. identification of the test item by code or name (IUPAC, CAS number, biological parameters, etc.)
     iii. identification of the reference item by name
     iv. characterization of the test item including purity, stability and homogeneity
    b. **Information concerning the sponsor and the test facility**
       i. name and address of the sponsor
      ii. name and address of any test facilities and test sites involved
     iii. name and address of the study director
     iv. name and address of any principal investigators and the phase of the study delegated, if applicable
      v. name and address of scientists having contributed reports to the final report
    c. **Dates**
      experimental starting and completion dates
    d. **Statement**
      a quality assurance programme statement listing the types of inspections made and their dates, including the phases inspected, and the dates any inspection results were reported to management and to the study director and any principal investigators, if applicable. This statement would also serve to confirm that the final report reflects the raw data
    e. **Description of materials and test methods**
       i. description of methods and materials used
      ii. reference to OECD test guidelines or other test guidelines or methods
    f. **Results**
       i. a summary of results
      ii. all information and data required in the study plan
     iii. a presentation of the results, including calculations and determinations of statistical significance
     iv. an evaluation and discussion of the results and, where appropriate, conclusions

g. **Storage**

the location where the study plan, samples of test and reference items, specimens, raw data and the final report are to be stored.

PART X

STORAGE AND RETENTION OF RECORDS AND MATERIALS

1. 1. The following should be retained in the archives for the period specified by the appropriate regulatory authorities -
   a. the study plan, raw data, samples of test and reference items, specimens and the final report of each regulatory study
   b. records of all inspections performed by the quality assurance programme, as well as master schedules
   c. records of qualifications, training, experience and job descriptions of personnel
   d. records and reports of the maintenance and calibration of apparatus
   e. validation documentation for computerized systems
   f. the historical file of all standard operating procedures
   g. environmental monitoring records
   2. In the absence of a required retention period, the final disposition of any study materials should be documented. When samples of test and reference items and specimens are disposed of before the expiry of the required retention period for any reason, this should be justified and documented. Samples of test and reference items and specimens should be retained only as long as the quality of the preparation permits evaluation.

2. Material retained in the archives should be indexed so as to facilitate orderly storage and retrieval.

3. Only personnel authorized by management should have access to the archives. Movement of material in and out of the archives should be properly recorded.

4. If a test facility or an archive contracting facility goes out of business and has no legal successor, the archive should be transferred to the archives of the sponsor of the regulatory study.

QCT-12.5

 Health Santé
Canada Canada

GOOD PRACTICES IN QUALITY CONTROL

17.1 Quality control is the part of GMP concerned with sampling, specifications and testing, and with the organization, documentation and release procedures which ensure that the necessary and relevant tests are actually carried out and that materials are not released for use, nor products released for sale or supply, until their quality has been judged to be satisfactory. Quality control is not confined to laboratory operations but must be involved in all decisions concerning the quality of the product.

17.2 The independence of quality control from production is considered fundamental.

17.3 Each manufacturer (the holder of a manufacturing authorization) should have a quality control function. The quality control function should be independent of other departments and under the authority of a person with appropriate qualifications and experience, who has one or several control laboratories at his or her disposal. Adequate resources must be available to ensure that all the quality control arrangements are effectively and reliably carried out. The basic requirements for quality control are as follows:

a. Adequate facilities, trained personnel and approved procedures must be available for sampling, inspecting, and testing starting materials, packaging materials, and intermediate, bulk, and finished products, and where appropriate for monitoring environmental conditions for GMP purposes.

b. Samples of starting materials, packaging materials, intermediate products, bulk products and finished products must be taken by methods and personnel approved of by the quality control department.

c. Qualification and validation must be performed.

d. Records must be made (manually and/or by recording instruments) demonstrating that all the required sampling, inspecting and testing procedures have actually been carried out and that any deviations have been fully recorded and investigated.

e. The finished products must contain ingredients complying with the qualitative and quantitative composition of the product described in the marketing authorization; the ingredients must be of the required purity, in their proper container and correctly labelled.

f. Records must be made of the results of inspecting and testing the materials and intermediate, bulk and finished products against specifications; product assessment must include a review and evaluation of the relevant production documentation and an assessment of deviations from specified procedures.

g. No batch of product is to be released for sale or supply prior to certification by the authorized person(s) that it is in accordance with the requirements of the marketing authorization. In certain countries, by law, the batch release is a task of the authorized person from production together with the authorized person from quality control.

h. Sufficient samples of starting materials and products must be retained to permit future examination of the product if necessary; the retained product must be kept in its final pack unless the pack is exceptionally large.

17.4 Quality control as a whole will also have other duties, such as to establish, validate and implement all quality control procedures, to evaluate, maintain, and store the reference standards for substances, to ensure the correct labelling of containers of materials and products, to ensure that the stability of the active pharmaceutical ingredients and products is monitored, to participate in the investigation of complaints related to the quality of the product, and to participate in environmental monitoring. All these operations should be carried out in accordance with written procedures and, where necessary, recorded.

17.5 Assessment of finished products should embrace all relevant factors, including the production conditions, the results of in-process testing, the manufacturing (including packaging) documentation, compliance with the specification for the finished product, and an examination of the finished pack.

17.6 Quality control personnel must have access to production areas for sampling and investigation as appropriate.

CONTROL OF STARTING MATERIALS AND INTERMEDIATE, BULK AND FINISHED PRODUCTS

17.7 All tests should follow the instructions given in the relevant written test procedure for each material or product. The result should be checked by the supervisor before the material or product is released or rejected.

17.8 Samples should be representative of the batches of material from which they are taken in accordance with the approved written procedure.

17.9 Sampling should be carried out so as to avoid contamination or other adverse effects on quality. The containers that have been sampled should be marked accordingly and carefully resealed after sampling.

17.10 Care should be taken during sampling to guard against contamination or mix-up of, or by, the material being sampled. All sampling equipment that comes into contact with the material should be clean. Some particularly hazardous or potent materials may require special precautions.

17.11 Sampling equipment should be cleaned and, if necessary, sterilized before and after each use and stored separately from other laboratory equipment.

17.12 Each sample container should bear a label indicating:
   a. The name of the sampled material
   b. The batch or lot number
   c. The number of the container from which the sample has been taken
   d. The number of the sample
   e. The signature of the person who has taken the sample
   f. The date of sampling

17.13 OOS results obtained during testing of materials or products should be investigated in accordance with an approved procedure. Records should be maintained.

TEST REQUIREMENTS

STARTING AND PACKAGING MATERIALS

17.14 Before releasing a starting or packaging material for use, the quality control manager should ensure that the materials have been tested for conformity with specifications for identity, strength, purity and other quality parameters.

17.15 An identity test should be conducted on a sample from each container of starting material (see also Section 14.14).

17.16 Each batch (lot) of printed packaging materials must be examined following receipt.

17.17 In lieu of testing by the manufacturer, a certificate of analysis may be accepted from the supplier, provided that the manufacturer establishes the reliability of the supplier's analysis through appropriate periodic validation of the supplier's test results (see Sections 8.8 and 8.9) and through on-site audits of the supplier's capabilities. (This does not affect Section 17.15.) Certificates must be originals (not photocopies) or otherwise have their authenticity assured. Certificates must contain at least the following information (6):
   a. Identification (name and address) of the issuing supplier
   b. Signature of the competent official, and statement of his or her qualifications
   c. The name of the material tested
   d. The batch number of the material tested

    e. The specifications and methods used

    f. The test results obtained

    g. The date of testing

IN-PROCESS CONTROL

17.18 In-process control records should be maintained and form a part of the batch records (see Section 15.25).

FINISHED PRODUCTS

17.19 For each batch of drug product, there should be an appropriate laboratory determination of satisfactory conformity to its finished product specification prior to release.

17.20 Products failing to meet the established specifications or any other relevant quality criteria should be rejected.

BATCH RECORD REVIEW

17.21 Production and quality control records should be reviewed as part of the approval process of batch release. Any divergence or failure of a batch to meet its specifications should be thoroughly investigated. The investigation should, if necessary, extend to other batches of the same product and other products that may have been associated with the specific failure or discrepancy. A written record of the investigation should be made and should include the conclusion and follow-up action.

17.22 Retention samples from each batch of finished product should be kept for at least one year after the expiry date. Finished products should usually be kept in their final packaging and stored under the recommended conditions. If exceptionally large packages are produced, smaller samples might be stored in appropriate containers. Samples of active starting materials should be retained for at least one year beyond the expiry date of the corresponding finished product. Other starting materials (other than solvents, gases, and water) should be retained for a minimum of two years if their stability allows.

Retention samples of materials and products should be of a size sufficient to permit at least two full re-examinations.

STABILITY STUDIES

17.23 Quality control should evaluate the quality and stability of finished pharmaceutical products and, when necessary, of starting materials and intermediate products.

17.24 Quality control should establish expiry dates and shelf-life specifications on the basis of stability tests related to storage conditions.

17.25 A written programme for ongoing stability determination should be developed and implemented to include elements such as:

   a. A complete description of the drug involved in the study

   b. The complete set of testing parameters and methods, describing all tests for potency, purity, and physical characteristics and documented evidence that these tests indicate stability

   c. Provision for the inclusion of a sufficient number of batches

   d. The testing schedule for each drug

   e. Provision for special storage conditions

   f. Provision for adequate sample retention

   g. A summary of all the data generated, including the evaluation and the conclusions of the study

17.26 Stability should be determined prior to marketing and following any significant changes in processes, equipment, packaging materials, and so on.

REFERENCES

1. Good manufacturing practices for pharmaceutical products. In: *WHO Expert Committee on Specifications for Pharmaceutical Preparations.* Twenty-second report. Geneva: World Health Organization, 1992, Annex 1 (WHO Technical Report Series, No. 823).

2. Validation of analytical procedures used in the examination of pharmaceutical materials. In: *WHO Expert Committee on Specifications for Pharmaceutical Preparations.* Thirty-second report. Geneva: World Health Organization, 1992, Annex 5 (WHO Technical Report Series, No. 823).

3. Good manufacturing practice for medicinal products in the European Community. Brussels, Commission of the European Communities, 1992. 4. Pharmaceutical Inspection Convention, Pharmaceutical Inspection Cooperation Scheme (PIC/S). In: *Guide to Good Manufacturing Practice for Medicinal Plants.* Geneva: PIC/S Secretariat, 2000.

5. Quality assurance of pharmaceuticals. *A Compendium of Guidelines and Related Materials. Volume 2. Good Manufacturing Practices and Inspection.* Geneva: World Health Organization, 1999.

6. Model certificate of analysis. In: *WHO Expert Committee on Specifications for Pharmaceutical Preparations.* Thirty-sixth report. Geneva: World Health Organization, 2002, Annex 10 (WHO Technical Report Series, No. 902).

Index